AF477232

BOOST YOUR METABOLISM DIET & COOKBOOK

The Little Metabolism Booster Diet Book for Weight Loss

BRITTNEY DAVIS

CRAIG WILLIAMS

Other Books By Brittney & Craig

- Liver Detox & Cleanse
- Gut Detox & Cleanse
- Carb Cycling Diet Plan & Cookbook

Contents

Recipes

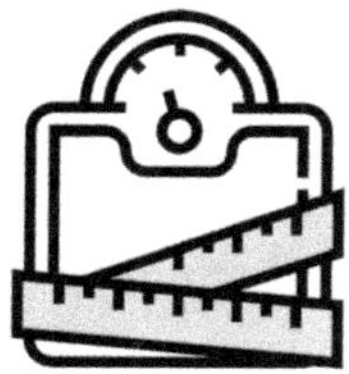

An Introduction to Your Metabolism

Remember when you were fifteen, and you could eat junk food every day and stay skinny? Maybe that continued into your twenties or even your thirties.

But at some point, you woke up and noticed that your clothes didn't fit anymore, and the tummy that used to be flat wasn't as tight anymore. Your habits hadn't noticeably changed, but the way your body responded to them sure did.

Most people will experience exactly this.

As we get older, our activity levels tend to drop, often slowly and unnoticeably. If, at the same time, we keep eating like we're teenagers without a care in the world, it will catch up with us. Unfortunately, even if you change your eating habits and try to keep up with exercise, very often, our metabolic rate changes as we get older.

It happens slowly, so you might not even notice that you're gaining a size every few years. Then, one day you wake up and realize that you have fifty pounds to lose and no idea where to start. So, you diet, but even that doesn't work as well as it used to, and at some point, you're left with a few stubborn pounds that just won't shift.

If you recognized yourself in this, you're in the right place.

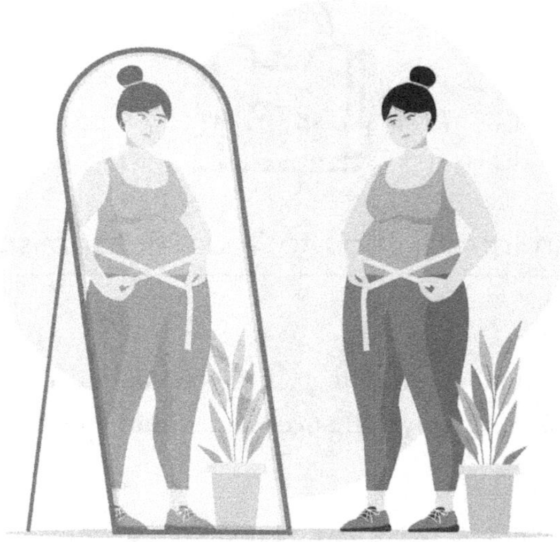

This book is all about metabolism. What it is, how it works, and more importantly, why it changes over time. It's also about how you can kickstart things and get your sluggish body burning fat faster again.

Middle-Aged Spread Is Real

You've probably heard the term "middle-aged spread." It's a term used to describe the weight many people tend to gain as they reach a certain age – usually from their mid to late thirties and upwards. It's a cliché because it happens so often.

This means that if you used to be able to inhale a pizza without gaining an ounce, you're not alone. There are scientific reasons for all of it, but that also means it's possible to use science to your advantage. If a slowing metabolic rate is to blame for your weight gain (and it usually is), then speeding up your metabolism is the solution.

While it may be common to gain weight as you age, it's not by any means inevitable. You also don't have to live a completely different lifestyle. But you will need to make a few tweaks to stay in shape!

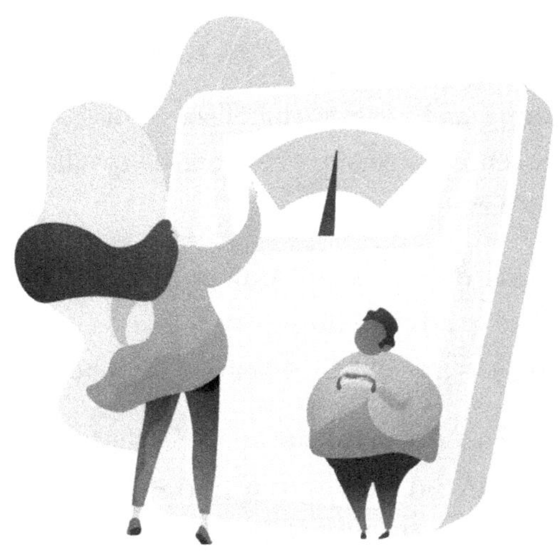

Weight That Just Won't Shift

The other thing that many people discover as they age is that while it is infinitely easier to gain weight, it becomes exponentially harder to lose it.

You used to be able to diet for a week or two and watch the pounds drop right off. Now you have to eat lettuce for a month just to lose one or two stubborn pounds.

That's likely all because of your metabolism. When we're younger, our metabolism burns fat and stored carbohydrates much faster, which means we can eat more and not gain weight, but also, if we reduce our caloric intake, we lose weight more quickly.

The older we get, and the more sluggish our metabolic rate becomes, the harder we have to work to shift weight and keep it off.

Harder to Stay the Course

When you're young and your metabolism is fast, it's a lot easier to stick to a diet – even a restrictive one. You see results quickly, and the weight stays off when you lose it.

But if you're staring down month four or five of eating like a rabbit, chances are you're ready to throw in the towel and replace your wardrobe with joggers and oversize items. That's normal.

The solution is not to cut more out of your diet. It's to change how your body processes food, so you can start eating a little more of the stuff you like. After all, if you know you can still have take-out for dinner once a week, it's a lot easier to stick to a diet the other six days!

What You Will Learn

The problem with many diets and weight loss plans is that they're built on mystery. Companies and weight loss gurus know that if they can keep you confused, they can keep taking your money, month after month.

This book is not one of those schemes.

In this book, we will give you all the facts so that you can create your own diet and lifestyle plan that works for you, and that you can stick to and adjust as needed.

You're going to learn exactly what metabolism actually is, how it works, why it stops working, and how you can get it started again. You're also going to learn what you did (without even knowing) that started the decline so that you can avoid it from now on.

There are also easy-to-follow recipes featured that you can use to create meals that you won't dread and give you all the tools you need to create a metabolism-friendly lifestyle.

More importantly, we're going to show you the difference between active weight loss and maintenance, and how you can moderate your metabolic rate, diet, and exercise to stay at your ideal weight and fitness level.

Why Me?

When I was a kid, my family used to tell me that I had hollow legs. I could literally eat everything and not gain an ounce. Of course, at the same time, I was swimming, roller skating, running, playing soccer, and working in active, demanding jobs.

My easy weight loss continued into my twenties and even after I had my first child.

But, life happens, and after a certain age, like most people, I stopped skating, running, swimming, and biking, and the pounds started to sneak on slowly. It's always slow too, so you never really seem to notice, until one day you look in the mirror and don't recognize yourself at all!

Of course, the first response is always to reach for the miracle pills and potions, but those mostly don't work either. So, I did what I always do – research.

Most of the secrets of a healthy lifestyle aren't secrets at all. They're biological facts that are well documented. You just have to know where to find them. But I've done that work for you, and this book will give you a foundation to build your healthy lifestyle plan on. So, you can get rid of that middle-aged spread, and get back to the look and feel you didn't appreciate nearly enough when you were younger!

Let's get to it!

CREATE HEALTHY HABITS, NOT RESTRICTIONS...

– Unknown

ONE

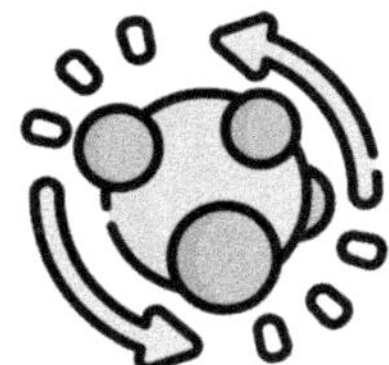

What exactly is metabolism?

Usually, when we think about biology, that's all we think about. But I like to think about metabolism in terms of a different kind of science. In this case, physics. Or, to be more specific, Isaac Newton's third law, which is one of the foundations of our knowledge of the world.

Newton said, "For every action, there is an equal and opposite reaction."

He was talking about matter and forces, but that's true of your body too.

Everything you do (or don't do) and every choice you make will have an effect on the way you look and feel. Maybe you won't notice it immediately, but it will.

In fact, over time, all those little actions and inactions are going to have some pretty significant effects! Which is probably why you're here right now!

So, we need to know more about how the "force" of your metabolism works.

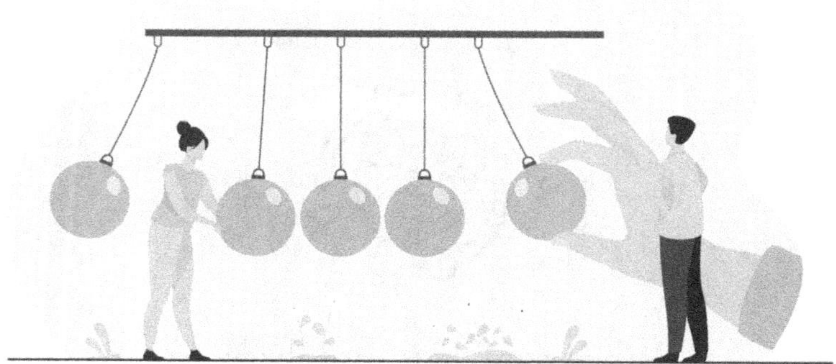

What Is Your Metabolism?

In very simple terms, your metabolism is the rate at which your body burns the calories (or energy) you get from food and drinks.

Think of your body like an engine. Or rather, a lot of very tiny engines (your cells) all working together to power an amazing amount of processes.

Like every engine, those cells require energy to function, and in this case, that energy comes from the things we eat and drink. If the energy we need matches the fuel we put into the system, there's no extra leftover. If we have too much fuel, your body has to pile it up somewhere.

Which is where body fat comes from. It's our personal fuel storage area.

There are a few parts to this process that we will look at in more detail in a moment: your basal metabolic rate, thermogenesis (or converting food to fuel for your cells), and physical activity, which increases the amount of fuel you need.

Each of those things will determine how much energy your body uses and what's leftover to go into storage!

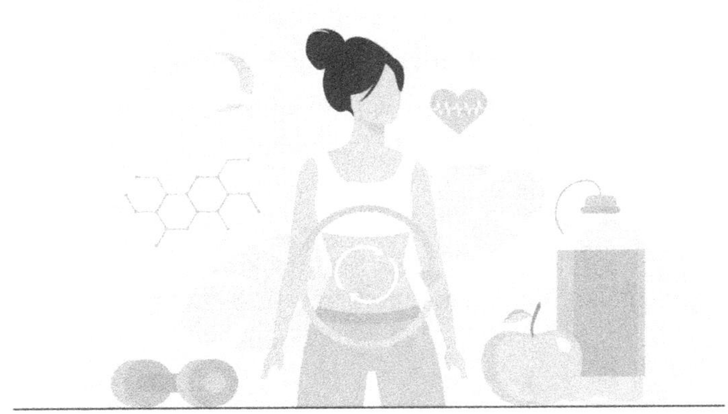

Your Basal Metabolic Rate

Your basal metabolic rate is what most people think of when they think of metabolism. This is the rate at which our bodies burn calories, even when we're doing nothing. Because even when you're sitting still or sleeping, your cells need energy. They just need a little less!

Most people have a higher basal metabolic rate when they are younger because most people are more active as children and teens. That means that we have more muscles and less fat, and muscle cells require more fuel to do what they do.

There are a few other factors that determine your basal metabolic rate too. Your overall body size is another one, because taller, heavier people burn more fuel than shorter, lighter ones. Your age is also a factor. Just like a twenty-year-old car loses fuel efficiency, your body loses a little metabolic rate as you age.

However, while some of those changes are unavoidable, some things can be done to increase your basal metabolic rate. This way, you can burn more fuel, even when you're not exercising. Luckily, it's not written in stone, and we are free to make changes for the better!

One easy way to increase your basal metabolic rate is to increase the proportion of muscle to fat in your body. This means working out can actually help you to lose more weight even when you're not trying!

Thermogenesis

Thermogenesis is a fancy name for digesting and processing the food you eat.

Like all of the processes in your body, this process burns fuel. In fact, for people who are eating a normal, healthy, and balanced diet, about 10% of the energy stored in the food you eat will be burned just by eating it!

This has given rise to terms like "negative calorie foods." These are foods where we burn more energy than they contain when you eat them.

While they're not exactly negative calories (and it doesn't cancel them out altogether), things like raw fruits and veggies fall into this category. Crunching through a carrot takes effort, which burns a higher percentage of the calories you're getting from them.

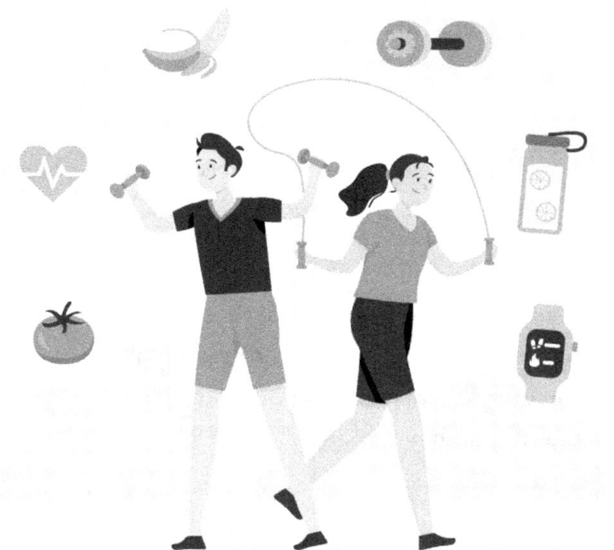

Physical Activity

Physical activity is the third pillar of your metabolism. If you're putting calories into the system, you need to be burning an equal amount to maintain your weight, or more if you want to lose weight.

If you eat more calories than you burn, through a combination of basal metabolic rate, thermogenesis, and physical activity, you're going to gain weight.

It's straightforward, and now you see why it reminds me of Newton!

A Simple Equation

As you can see so far, metabolism is a pretty simple concept. There are no magic pills or potions that can speed up your metabolism, but there are simple things you can do to change the result of the equation.

If you reduce the number of calories you consume, increase your physical activity, and change the ratio of muscle to fat in your body, you will literally tip the scales in your favor.

Now that you know the equation and what you can control, it's time to take a closer look at how you can make those changes. Better still, you can make those changes in ways that are sustainable and in ways you can live with every day. Because no one can live on a restrictive diet forever, nor should you have to!

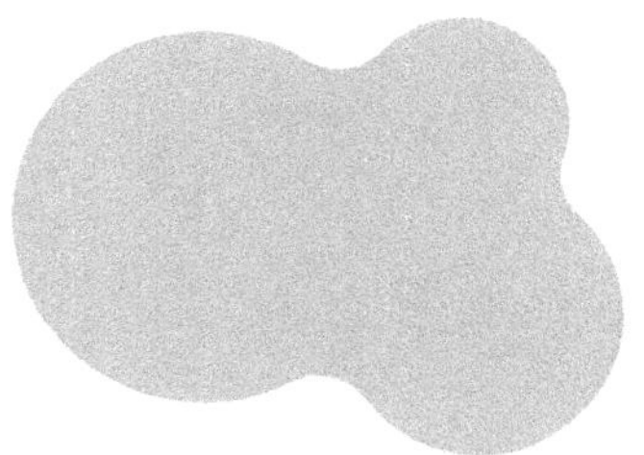

WHAT YOU WANT IS TO REV UP YOUR METABOLISM SO THAT YOU ARE BURNING FAT AND CALORIES, NOT PRESERVING FAT AND CALORIES.

– Kathy Freston

TWO

State of Today

Globally, we're getting heavier.

In fact, since 1980, the number of obese people on the planet has doubled in over seventy countries. Over 600 million adults (or more than 12 percent), and over 107 million children (or over 5 percent), are clinically obese.

This is despite all of our ever-expanding knowledge about health and wellness, better access to nutritious food, and many other factors.

Weight-related diseases like diabetes, heart disease, certain types of weight-related cancer, and others are all on the rise.

But it's not all because we're choosing junk food. The global increase in obesity and unhealthy weight gain is not all about the "meal" choices we make. In fact, many of the reasons we're struggling like this are direct side effects of our *lifestyle*.

That's not that surprising. But what might surprise you is that not all of the reasons for our global weight loss are food-related. In fact, there are several things aside from what we eat that can have a marked effect on weight gain.

Because a higher percentage of fat burns fewer calories than muscle, weight gain itself can slow down your metabolism. Weight gain also makes it harder to get moving, which also slows down your metabolic rate.

Of course, you still have to watch what you eat, but while you do, you need to pay attention to these lifestyle factors too.

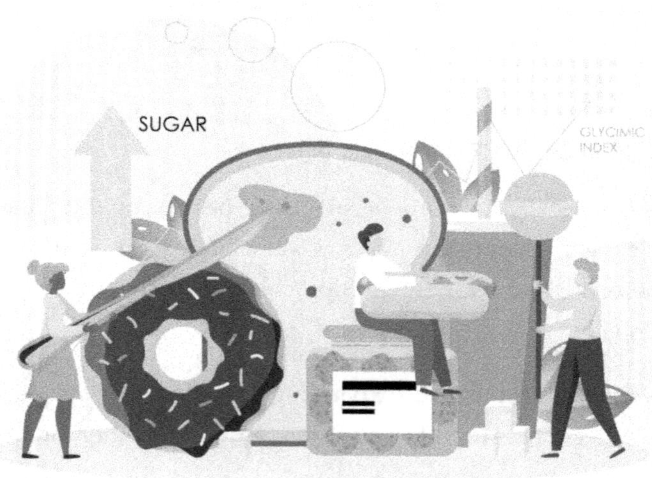

What We Eat

The first factor in any discussion about metabolism and weight gain has to be food. But, again, it's not all about the food itself.

Our lives are busier than ever. Jobs, hobbies, kids, studies, and many other things demand our time, so we turn to processed and convenience foods. They're quick. They're easy, and they give us more time to spend on all the other things that demand our attention.

But reaching for prepared foods is one of the worst things you can do for your health. It should be the exception rather than the rule.

The occasional trip to the drive-through or a box of ready-made chicken nuggets when you just don't have time won't derail your health. But you do need to make healthy choices 90 percent of the time.

Choose foods that are as close to their natural state as possible, prepare them yourself, and use healthier cooking methods like grilling or steaming. If you make a conscious effort to do that most of the time, you can still get away with a few treats.

We'll get into details and recipes soon, but for now, commit to reading food labels when you buy prepared foods, cook most of your food yourself, and choose fresh products.

Stress

We've all heard the term "stress eating." Some people call it "eating your feelings." Whatever you call it, it's more than just words. There's a direct link between stress and weight gain, both in terms of what we eat and the chemicals in our bodies. These make it easier to gain weight and more challenging to lose it.

About 30% of adults suffer from the effects of stress, and again, a lot of it is unavoidable. Jobs, kids, busy lives, financial pressure, relationship problems. They all cause us stress, and we've got less time than ever to address them in a healthy manner.

Chemically, stress has a profound hidden effect on our bodies, and one of the worst culprits is cortisol. Also known as the "stress hormone."

We produce and release this hormone in large quantities when we are stressed. It's part of the body's "fight or flight" mechanism. That's biologically supposed to trigger precisely that. But we can't fight the people who cause us stress at the office or in our lives, and we can't run away from our financial troubles. So, we stay stressed, and we eat our feelings.

Worse than that, cortisol triggers a release of insulin, and insulin makes us crave sugary, fatty foods. There's a reason they call it comfort food!

So, we're eating more to make ourselves feel better about stress, and we're eating all the wrong things because we're chemically craving them. That's a recipe for metabolic disaster!

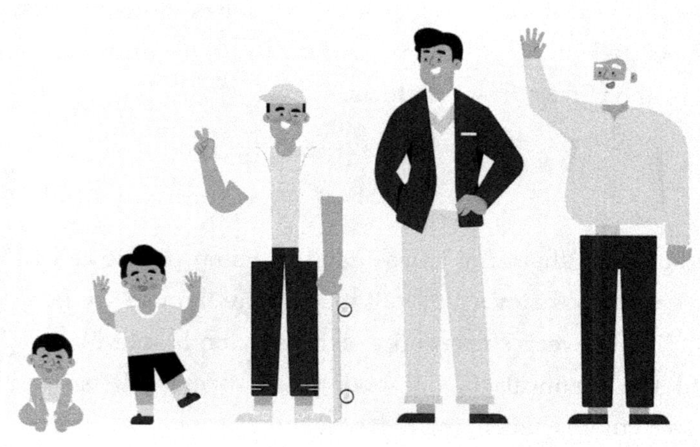

Aging

We've already touched on how aging tends to make some people less active. But even if your eating and exercise habits haven't changed, your biology may be against you.

There is a process in the body called "lipid turnover," which is related to how fat is stored and burned. As we age, this process slows down. So even people who don't eat more as they get older and stay active tend to gain weight.

In fact, in some studies, 20% of older adults who don't reduce their calory intake will gain weight, even if their lifestyle does not change in any other way.

This isn't great news, because it means that we have to adjust our lifestyle as we get older so that we can maintain the same level of health. But the good news is that while diet can keep your weight stable, there are signs that exercise may reverse the problem.

So, if you're not moving already, you need to get started, and instead of slowing down as you age, you need to increase your activity levels.

Too Much Dieting

Sounds strange, doesn't it? But dieting too much can actually slow down your metabolism and trigger your body to store more of the food you eat.

When you eat too little to keep yourself healthy (or dramatically change your eating habits quickly), your body assumes that you are starving.

When we are in a state of starvation, our bodies basically turn off what they think are non-essential processes and conserve as many calories as possible. Unfortunately, besides storing more of the food you do eat as fat, your body also turns off the systems that you need.

Like your immune system. Which means you might get sick easier.

Even if you do manage to eat so few calories that you lose weight, as your body weight decreases, so do both your energy levels and your metabolic rate. You're smaller, so you have fewer cells burning energy and fewer stores of energy available for exercise and activity.

When you return to eating a more normal diet, you may find that you gain weight much faster and struggle to lose it.

This is why crash diets are not only dangerous but bad for weight loss, and why so many people are yo-yo dieters. No one can sustain this kind of starvation diet, and while you're on it, you're actually making it harder to be healthy in the future.

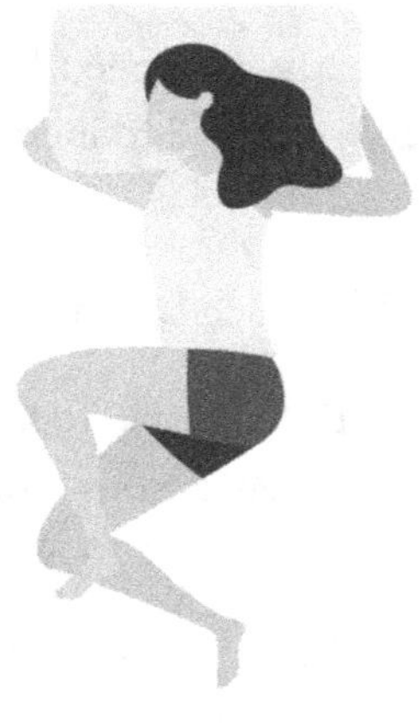

Sleep Habits

As if it wasn't bad enough that our eating habits, exercise habits, busy lives, and biology work against our metabolism, there's another factor. *Sleep*.

While we're trying to cram extra hours into the day, something has to give, and very often, that means sacrificing sleep. But research has shown that the less we sleep, the worse our metabolism is likely to perform.

Not only that, but a lack of sleep is tied to two chemicals, called ghrelin and leptin, which control our appetite.

The less sleep you get, the hungrier you are likely to be, and the more you are likely to crave calorie-dense, carbohydrate-high foods. At the same time, because you're tired and dealing with unpaid sleep debt, you're likely to have less energy. This means you are far less likely to get out and get moving.

So, if you're not sleeping enough, and it goes on for too long, it's going to start showing on the scale.

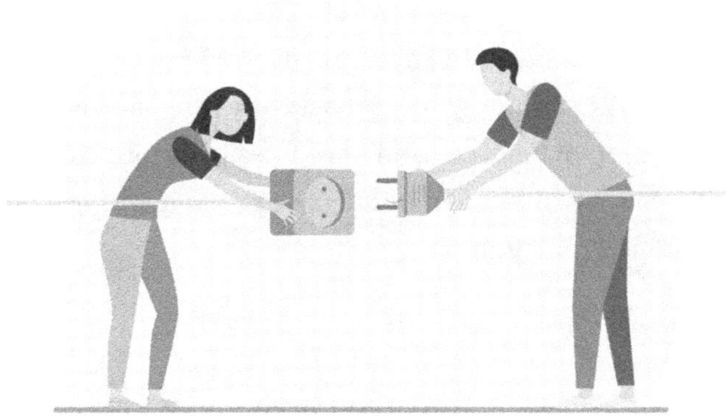

Everything Is Connected

When we think of weight loss and even metabolism, we tend to think of food and exercise, and leave it at that.

But our bodies are incredibly complex bio-electrical machines that have thousands of complex processes happening all the time.

Everything we do or don't do has an impact on our health and on our weight and fitness. You cannot make major, lasting changes to your metabolic rate or waistline without changing everything you do.

If you've been struggling to lose weight and keep it off, then that's the first thing you need to consider. Are you only doing some of the things you need to improve your health?

Are you letting your stress levels rise unchecked and spending sleepless nights because of it? You probably won't get the results you want. Are you trying to cut out too many calories so you don't have to exercise? It won't work. At least, not in the long term.

Before you continue reading, it might be worth examining your life as a whole and look for all the areas that you might need to work on to get your overall health under control. Calorie restrictive diets alone will not be enough to get your metabolism working correctly and keep the pounds off. As soon as you go back to eating normally, you will simply put the weight back on, and very possibly more. You might also drive your metabolic rate down in the process, so it will be even harder to lose weight next time you try.

**EVEN THE SMALLEST
CHANGES IN OUR DAILY
ROUTINE CAN CREATE
INCREDIBLE RIPPLE EFFECTS
THAT EXPAND OUR VISION
OF WHAT IS POSSIBLE.**

– Charles F. Glassman

THREE

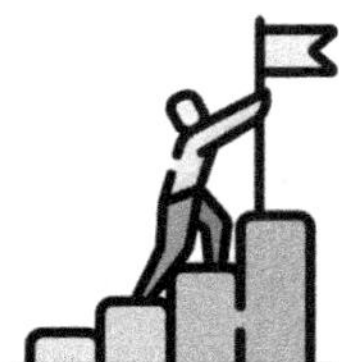

Basics of Improving Metabolism

Now that you know what your metabolism is, what it does, and what can affect it, the next logical question is what you can do to make it work harder. The faster your metabolism works, the easier it is to lose weight and stay in shape.

But you've probably also realized that your metabolism, like other processes in your body, is complex. Everything that happens in our bodies is a network of processes, chemicals, and more. It's all interconnected, and there are usually many different factors involved.

This is why most of the pills, potions, and miracle weight loss promises out there don't work. Most of them focus on only one or two elements of weight loss, health, and fitness, and even if they work, they could throw everything out of balance. That means that they might even cause more problems than they solve.

The good news is that once you understand all of this and realize that there are many different issues to address, you can start working on all of them.

The Basics

As you've seen, while food and exercise are essential to our health, you also need to address many other, secondary factors if you want to improve your metabolism. These include:

- Your diet. While it's certainly not the only thing that affects your metabolism, you do need to have enough calories (but not too much) and get your calories from the right kinds of foods.
- Exercise, which both burns more calories immediately and converts fat into muscle. Muscle burns more calories than other types of cells.
- Stress management. There are far too many adverse effects and chemicals related to stress. If you are suffering from stress in your life, particularly long-term or unavoidable stress, you should find ways to deal with and minimize it.
- Address sleep problems. Sleep is closely tied to every aspect of your health – including your metabolism!

Any weight loss program that doesn't address your whole life is unlikely to succeed in the long term. If you don't fix or change all of the factors that impact your metabolism and make holistic lifestyle changes, you risk being stuck in a cycle of yo-yo dieting.

What Affects Your Metabolism?

You know you have to take a holistic approach to improving your metabolism. You know several factors might affect your ability to lose weight now and keep it off. You've learned that the things you do can speed up and slow down your metabolism.

But it's a good idea to take a closer look at some of these factors, so you can figure out what you should focus on and what you can let slide.

Your Age

You can stay in shape. Wear sunscreen. Get a facelift. You can dye your hair to hide the grey and whiten your teeth. But even if you look twenty years younger on the outside, you can't fool father time!

As we age, there are biological changes in our bodies. The chemicals and hormones we produce change, and that triggers other changes.

One of those changes will be in your metabolism. It will naturally slow down, to a greater or lesser degree, for everyone. A variety of factors come into play here, though, including what kind of shape you were, to begin with.

However, while you can't stop the biological process of aging, which doesn't mean you should throw your hands up in the air, sit on the couch and eat all the cookies! If you make changes to your lifestyle as your body rearranges itself, you can keep pace with the differences and still stay in great shape.

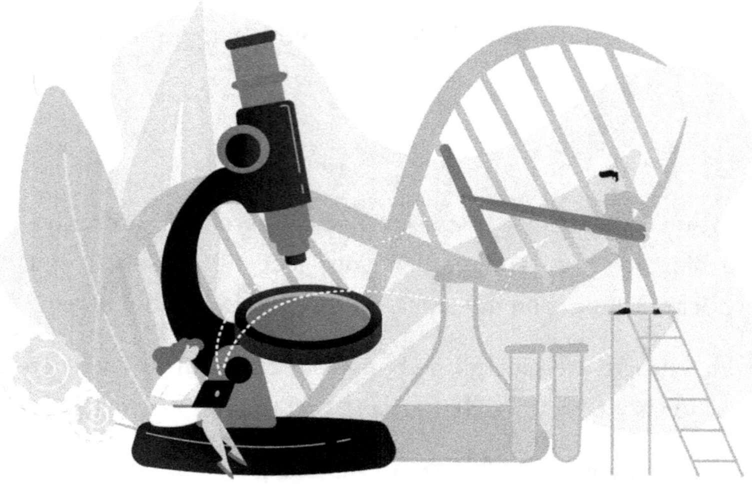

Genetics

Some people are naturally tall and slender, graceful and sporty. Then there are people who are naturally short and gain weight if they look at a cookie – and everyone in between.

We can't control our genetics or how they affect the chemicals and processes in our bodies. But we can pay attention to how our genetics predispose us to react to food and exercise and build our lifestyle around them.

So, if you know you gain weight when you look at a cookie, plan your week's activities, so you can feel like you deserve some. Don't give up the things you really want. Just make adjustments that make them less of a problem.

Weight and Body Type

Your weight and body type (particularly the ratio of fat to muscle) is a massive part of how well or otherwise poor your metabolism works. But it's not only about being overweight.

As we've already discussed, if you weigh too little or regularly starve yourself to lose weight, you can actually cause your metabolic rate to drop. So, when you go back to eating normally, and your body is still in starvation mode, you actually gain weight much faster.

There are risks to being both under and overweight, and messing with your metabolism is one of them.

To be generally healthy, you should aim for a BMI of between 18.5 and 24.9 and try to keep your body fat between 8% and 19% for men and 21% to 33% for women.

Believe it or not, your weight is one of the easier metabolism factors to control. But remember that other factors may affect your weight.

Before you blame your metabolism or even your diet or lifestyle for weight loss, you should consider other possibilities.

Many health conditions, including thyroid conditions, PCOS (polycystic ovarian syndrome), and many others, can result in hormonal imbalances. This, along with other conditions, can cause increased weight gain.

If you are eating a healthy diet, are doing moderate exercise, and are still gaining weight, you may first need to consult your doctor to rule out any potential underlying problems. Most of these conditions can be treated through lifestyle changes and medication if necessary. Once those adjustments are made, it will probably be easier to lose weight and get your metabolism back on track.

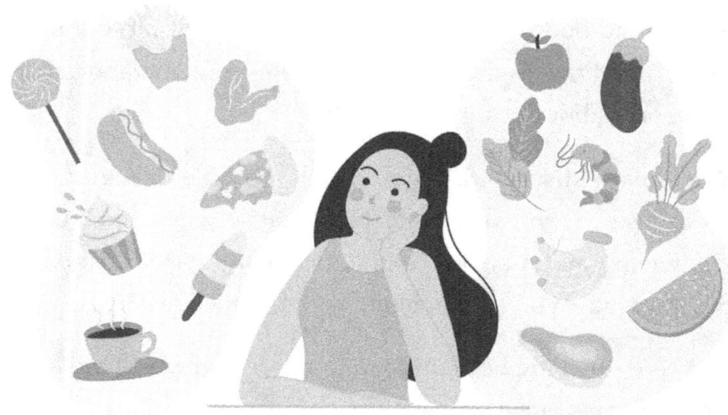

Diet

Your diet is one of the biggest things that you do control. Choosing whole foods, cooking them yourself using healthier cooking methods, and avoiding junk food is a good start. But there are other dietary choices you can make to improve your metabolism.

One way to do that is to choose low GI foods, which take longer to digest and don't create significant blood sugar spikes that can affect your energy levels and leave you starving when it drops again.

Another good idea is to break your daily eating habits into six smaller meals rather than the more conventional three. Again, this helps keep your blood sugar stable, which keeps you from being ravenous when you eat. If you're not entirely starving when you eat, you will eat more slowly and are less likely to overeat.

Then there's the popular option of restricting carbs. Eating fewer carbs and more protein, fat, and vegetables is an excellent way to fuel muscle and encourage fat burning. Because muscle burns more calories than fat, this can help to increase your metabolism.

There are many ways you can tweak what you eat, and even when you eat it, that have an impact on your metabolism. Research has found that even eating breakfast can change how your body processes food for the rest of the day.

So, take some time to think consciously about what you eat, when you eat it, and how it is prepared. Make better choices, but don't forget to allow the occasional cheat. No one can live on bland, boring food all the time. Don't torture yourself!

Exercise

Aside from diet, one of the things we have the most control over when it comes to metabolism, health, and weight loss, is exercise.

If exercise is a dirty word to you, though, or you immediately have visions of hours spent sweating in the gym, don't be discouraged!

Yes, gyms are an excellent place to work out, but they're not your only option. Team sports, whether it's a weekend soccer league with your friends in the park or something a little more formal, are also a great, fun way to get fitter.

If you don't like team sports, there are plenty of solo activities you can try too. Skating, running, or biking are fun by yourself or with a friend. Swimming is another great choice, and because it's low impact, it's great if you have joint trouble too.

Even fun activities like dancing or learning skills like martial arts can help get you in better shape. Consider activities you already enjoy and can commit to doing three or four times a week for at least half an hour. Even a walk in the park with your dog counts!

In fact, while there's some doubt about the trend of hitting 10,000 steps a day to stay fit, if you love walking, get yourself a digital pedometer or smartwatch, and push yourself to walk a few kilometers a day.

Finally, while cardio is great for building up a sweat and losing weight, remember that muscle burns more calories than other types of tissue. So, spending some time each week on strength training like weight training or using resistance band-based exercise machines is a great idea too.

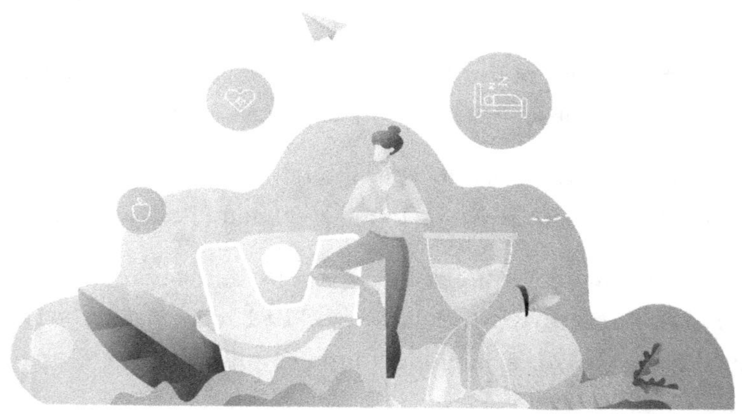

Lifestyle

Finally, there's your lifestyle. Diet, exercise, and your general health are a big part of that, but there are other things you can do to improve your metabolism.

Since stress is a significant factor in weight gain, it's a good idea to address anything that is causing stress in your life.

It's not possible to eliminate all the things that cause us stress. But you can learn to manage it better. Avoid using alcohol or other substances to cope. Consider things that you can do to reduce stress and do them. This is not only important for your metabolism but also for your overall health.

As we've already mentioned, sleep is another lifestyle factor that you may be surprised to find has a big impact on your metabolism. Both directly and indirectly, by making you less inclined to exercise.

Sleep is often tied to stress, so make sure you tackle that first. But when you have, you should be aiming to have at least seven hours of sleep every night and a regular sleep schedule. We will go into more detail about some strategies you can implement, but if you genuinely have trouble sleeping, speak to your doctor. Many options can help, but you have to ask to get them.

Everything is connected, and it's up to you to take the steps necessary to stay healthy.

Major Players

Lifestyle is a big part of controlling your metabolism, managing your weight, and staying healthy. But it's not the only factor.

Often, the choices we make trigger the creation or oversupply of chemicals in our bodies. Sometimes, they're the cause of metabolic trouble. If you are already taking care of the lifestyle factors we've mentioned, and you still struggle to control your weight, one of these might be the cause.

Once lifestyle factors are ruled out, your doctor can help you identify other possible causes of metabolic problems. If you want to treat the symptom (poor metabolism and weight gain), you will probably have to treat the cause first.

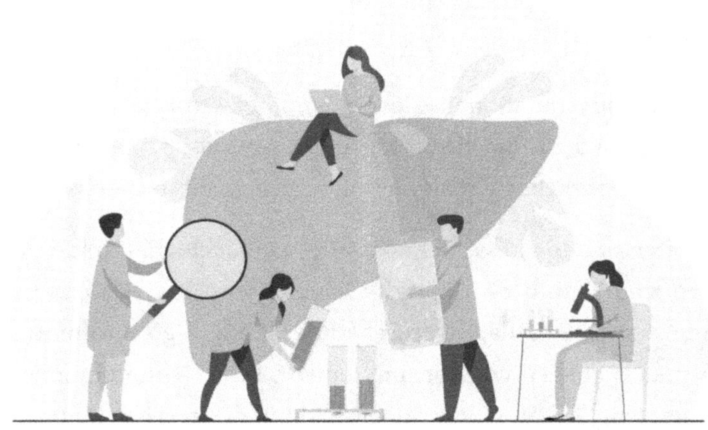

Liver

You probably don't think about your liver much, if at all. It's not usually something we think about. But when it comes to your metabolism, few organs in your body are as directly involved in the process.

Your liver converts nutrients from the food we eat into chemicals our cells can use. It also stores nutrients, including glycogen, which is a form of sugar that the liver gets from processing carbohydrates. When your blood sugar drops, the liver releases glycogen, which means it is also directly involved in regulating insulin. This is key, as your blood sugar and insulin levels determine when you will want to eat, and sometimes even what you want to eat!

Your diet has a significant impact on how well your liver works. Still, other factors like alcohol or drug use (even prescription drugs) can all play a role. Some people also have genetic conditions that cause their liver not to work as well as it should.

Liver conditions can be severe or even deadly, so if you suspect you might have any liver conditions, speak to your doctor.

Adrenals

Your adrenals are two glands that are found directly above your kidneys. They produce hormones that help regulate the processes in our bodies. One of those is aldosterone, which helps regulate blood pressure. Another one is cortisol, which is directly involved in your metabolism.

Your adrenal glands are also directly related to stress, which you might recognize from their role in creating *adrenaline*. So, when it comes to "fight or flight" and all the things that go with it, this is ground zero.

There are two parts to the adrenal glands – the cortex and the medulla. While both manufacture hormones we need to be healthy and survive, the most important one's come from the adrenal cortex.

Some of those hormones and chemicals are known as glucocorticoids. In the case of your metabolism, the most important is Hydrocortisone. Also known as cortisol, it regulates the conversions of protein, fat, and carbs into energy, among other things. In that way, it is literally one of the key players in metabolism.

As with your liver, you might not even know what your adrenals do, but they are critical to your health. If you have any concerns about your kidneys or adrenals, it's critical that you seek medical advice. There are severe conditions like Addison's disease and Cushing's disease that can affect your adrenals.

Thyroid

Your thyroid is another gland that creates and regulates hormones in your body. In this case, one of the primary functions of the thyroid is your metabolism.

Hypothyroidism is a condition where your thyroid doesn't create enough hormones, and your metabolism slows down. It's also known as an underactive thyroid. This can also cause thyroid hormones to drop to potentially dangerously low levels, known as myxedema.

Signs of an underactive thyroid (aside from metabolic issues) include:

- Low body temperature
- Heart failure
- Anemia
- Confusion and even coma

As you can see, an underactive thyroid is a lot more serious than just not being able to lose weight or keep it off. If you suspect you have thyroid problems, you should consult your doctor as soon as possible.

There is a blood test called a thyroid-stimulating hormone (TSH) test that can diagnose the condition. Medications like levothyroxine can increase the amount of thyroid hormone your body produces, improving your metabolism and keeping you healthy.

Do not ignore concerns about your thyroid. Left untreated, thyroid conditions can be dangerous or even deadly.

Pituitary Gland

The pituitary gland is another gland, this time in the brain, which controls various things like growth, reproduction, and metabolism.

The pituitary gland is actually known as the "master gland" because it produces some important hormones on its own. It also produces some that trigger other glands, like the adrenals.

Some of the hormones that your pituitary gland produces that are important to metabolism are:

- adrenocorticotropic hormone, which controls the secretion of cortisol by the adrenals.
- growth hormone, which is instrumental in growth, but also metabolism and body composition.
- thyroid-stimulating hormone, which helps to trigger your thyroid to make the thyroid hormones you need.

If you have hormonal problems, they may be related to the pituitary gland, and there are conditions like Cushing's and even tumors that may throw your hormone balance out of whack. These can be serious, so if you are experiencing metabolic problems and any other worrying symptoms, again, always consult your doctor.

Body Composition

As we have mentioned before, your metabolic rate will depend on many factors, including your body composition.

If you have a large amount of body fat and not as much muscle, you will burn calories slower. If you have more muscle, you will burn fat faster.

This is why, when you plan your exercise and activity, it's important to balance fat-burning activities like cardio with strength training, which, among other things, builds muscle.

WHILE WEIGHT LOSS IS IMPORTANT, WHAT'S MORE IMPORTANT IS THE *QUALITY* OF FOOD YOU PUT IN YOUR BODY – FOOD IS *INFORMATION* THAT QUICKLY CHANGES YOUR METABOLISM AND GENES.

– Mark Hyman

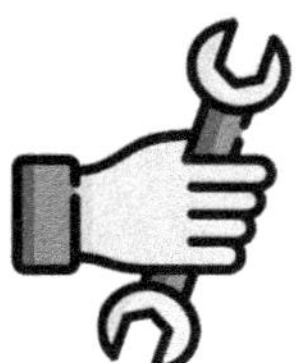

FOUR

Repairing Metabolic Damage Naturally

There are many products, pills, and potions out there that promise a rapid increase in your metabolic rate. They claim that they will get your body burning fat like a well-oiled machine. But the truth is, there are no magic pills out there, and you certainly wouldn't be able to buy them on the internet if there were!

There are some medications that can treat specific problems (like hypothyroidism) that could slow your metabolism. If you are diagnosed with one of those problems and given a prescription, that may increase your metabolism.

But, if you've been steadily gaining weight over several years, and your activity levels and diet are not exactly great, there's still more work to do.

The good news is that even if you have made choices that slowed your metabolism, there are still things you can do, naturally, to reverse the damage. Most of these are not complicated or costly.

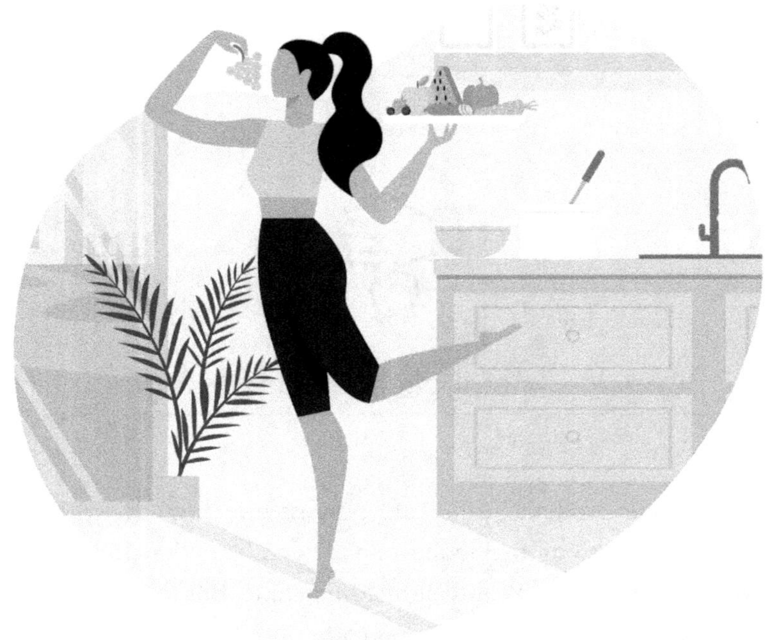

Change Your Eating Habits

You already know that you need to change what you eat if you want to lose weight, but there's more to it than just cutting calories.

First, as we've already discussed, avoid extreme diets. Yes, you may see short-term results, but you will slow your metabolism further, and as soon as you go back to normal eating, you will gain all the weight back.

Metabolism and weight loss are, as you might already have gathered, as much about regulating hormones and blood sugar as it is about cutting calories. A lot of that is simpler than you think.

- Choose high fiber foods and avoid processed white flour and sugar, which will cause your blood sugar to spike and trigger an insulin response.
- Eat healthy fats and protein, which will keep you fuller for longer, and, in the case of proteins, which fuel muscle cell production.
- Eat six small meals instead of three larger ones, spread out throughout the day, and make sure you balance carbs, fat, and protein.
- Drink more water, particularly cold water, before meals. Some studies show that this not only helps you eat less but may also stimulate thermogenesis, which burns more calories!
- Choose foods that take more energy to eat – like crunchy apples, other fruits, and veggies. It may not be much, but just the act of chewing and digesting them burns more calories.

A balanced diet is the basis of healthy weight loss and maintenance. Still, there are other "tricks" like these that can help your metabolism get the job done more efficiently.

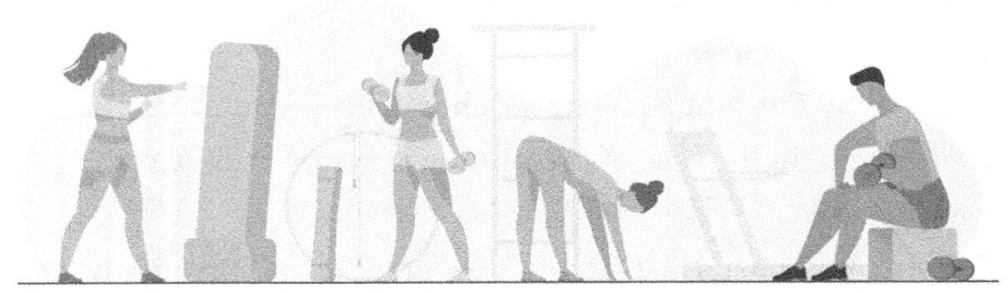

Build Muscle

We've said it before, but it bears repeating: muscle burns more calories.

Strength training, along with more lean protein in your diet, will help you build muscle and increase your body's fat-burning potential. Still, there are other benefits to weight or strength training.

Strength training improves bone density, which is particularly important for women, especially as they age. But it's a good thing for everyone else too!

Building muscle, particularly in your core, can also help relieve conditions like chronic back pain and improve mobility. This means you will be more able (and inclined) to work out, which in turn will help with losing weight and speeding up your metabolism.

Like other types of exercise, strength training also releases endorphins (or feel-good chemicals), so they improve your mood too!

If you're worried about turning into an overly muscled hulk, don't be! It takes a tremendous amount of weight training with concrete goals to even get close to that! A few hours of weight training a week will never get you to that!

Here are a few easy and affordable ways to incorporate weight training into your routine:

- Invest in a home gym. Most include various weight settings and resistance levels, and you can often get them much cheaper if you buy second hand!
- Buy yourself a set of dumbbells. They're very affordable, almost indestructible, come in various weight options, and are portable!
- Do "bodyweight" exercises, which use your own body weight. These include squats, push-ups, lunges, crunches, and similar.
- Try resistance bands. They're affordable, come in different resistance levels, and can be used in many different ways.

You don't need a gym membership or a personal trainer to get started with strength training. In fact, even a couple of full water bottles can be used if you don't have weights on hand. So, start today, and make a conscious effort to work on building muscle.

HIIT Workouts

HIIT or **High Intensity Interval Training** has become one of the most popular fitness choices in recent years, and it's relatively easy to get started.

HIIT is a workout consisting of a series of high-intensity exercises, interspersed with periods of rest. During the high-intensity part of the training, you will push yourself as hard and fast as you can go, which encourages your body to burn glucose.

Often, the period of activity is actually shorter than the recovery period during a HIIT workout. So you might sprint for 20 seconds and then rest for 40, before moving on to the next high-intensity activity.

This isn't just for running, though. You could do most kinds of aerobic exercise as HIIT, as long as you push yourself about as hard as you can go for a short time, and rest in between. Even cycling could be modified to be a HIIT workout. So instead of a long, leisurely ride, you would do intermittent bouts of high-speed riding, followed by a short rest, and then back to riding fast and hard. Push-ups, air squats, most exercises you can think of, can all be modified to fit into a HIIT workout.

HIIT was developed for athletes, and it's a great cardio choice. It also has other benefits, like improving cell insulin sensitivity and improves your heart function and blood pressure.

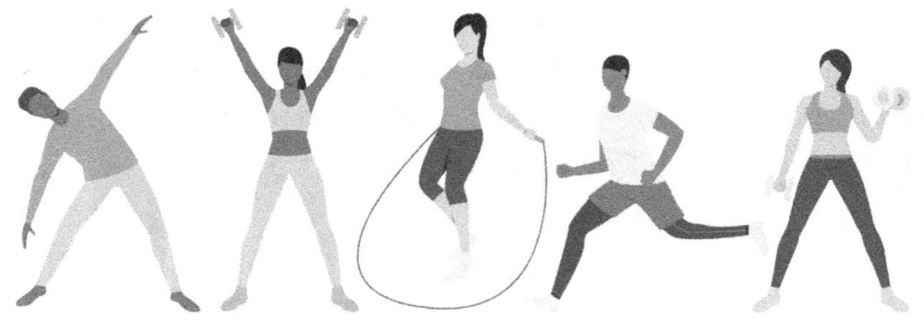

Focus on Moving!

It's been said that a sedentary lifestyle is the new smoking. While that might seem extreme, not moving enough can be almost as harmful to your heart and other systems.

Fortunately, unlike smoking, it's easy to undo the damage and to make the change from being a couch potato to getting back in shape. Here are a few simple tips you can try:

- Walk the dog. If you have a dog, taking her/him for a half an hour walk every day will make the little good boy/girl very happy and get you back on the road to fitness.
- Invest in a smartwatch and count your steps. While the 10,000 steps per day number is mostly arbitrary, if you walk that many steps every day, you will undoubtedly be fitter!
- Park further away from the grocery store when you go shopping. Yes, it's not much, but the extra walk is an easy way to build more movement into your day!
- Take the kids to the playground and join in! Kids are masters of movement, so see if you can keep up!
- Sign up for dance classes and go dancing once a week. Dancing is an excellent form of exercise!
- Take the stairs instead of the elevator if it's only a few floors. Or, if you have stairs at home, climb up and down them a few times a day to work your muscles and get your heart pumping.
- Clean your house. Housework is a surprisingly good workout, so skip the cleaning service and do it yourself. You will have a clean place, save money, and get fitter!

There are endless little things you can do every day to add more movement to your routine. Whether it's walking to the corner store instead of driving or a workout video in your basement while the kids are doing their homework, you can do it! Gym memberships are not required to get fit. Start small, be consistent, and keep improving, and you will be amazed at the results!

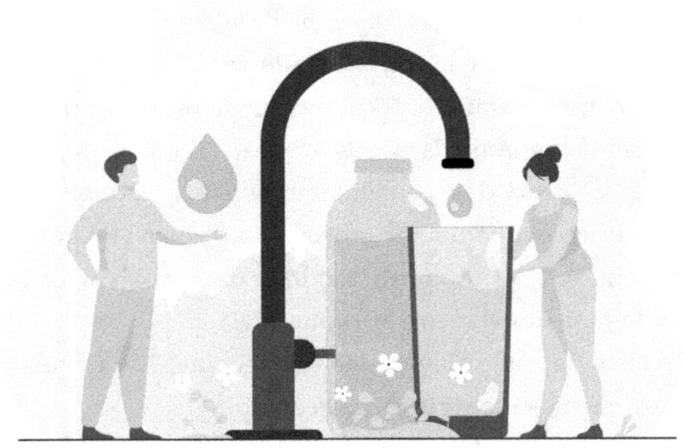

Drink Water

We've already touched on some of the ways that water can help you lose weight. Still, there are actually several more reasons why staying hydrated may be great for your metabolism.

It's an Appetite Suppressant.

Drinking water before you eat a meal has been shown to curb overeating because your stomach is already partially full of water when you start the meal. It takes a while before we know that we're full of the food we're eating, which means we may overeat before we even realize it. By drinking water before you eat, you limit the chance of that happening. In fact, studies show that drinking two small glasses of water before you eat can mean you eat 20% less or more.

It's a Metabolism Booster.

We've already mentioned that drinking cold water before a meal can improve your metabolic rate by triggering thermogenesis.

Cold water does this by forcing your body to expend energy heating the water to body temperature. Doing that requires energy, and energy comes from stored fat or from the calories we eat. Either way, it's good for weight loss!

Water is the Calorie-Free Choice!

We all know staying hydrated is essential, but there are so many choices! Soft drinks, juice, coffee, tea, and many more. Unlike water, however, most of those have calories in them.

Even when we're on a "diet", we tend not to count calories from liquids. This means that we might be consuming hundreds or even more calories every day than we need simply because of our drinks.

If you drink water, you won't be thirsty, and you won't be tempted by that pumpkin spice latte or anything else!

It Moves Electrolytes Around our Bodies.

Drinking water during exercise is vital to keeping us hydrated, but it's also important to help distribute electrolytes around our bodies.

To keep our muscles functioning properly when we exercise, we need to have various substances like sodium and potassium, which help our cells create the electrical energy they need to contract. Muscle contraction is movement in its simplest form.

Water helps to move those electrolytes around the body to where they are needed, making it easier for our muscles to work.

Water also cools us down and lets us cool ourselves during exercise by sweating. This helps prevent overheating, which can be dangerous. Basically, if you're going to be working out, you need to have more water than usual!

It's a Waste Remover.

Often, we forget that it's not just a matter of putting the right things in our bodies – we also have to make sure we get rid of waste!

If you don't drink enough water, you may not be able to get rid of enough toxins through urine or when you have a bowel movement.

Urine needs water to be adequately diluted, so that it doesn't burn or otherwise irritate you when you go to the bathroom. Water also helps flush out all the things that your kidneys have taken out of your bloodstream.

As for bowel movements, if you don't have enough water, you risk being constipated. Not only will that make you feel bloated, but no one feels like exercising when they're all backed up!

Water is Needed for Fat Burning.

We all know that fires require oxygen to burn, but did you know that your body needs water to burn fat?

The process of burning fat, which is known as lipolysis, actually decreases when we are dehydrated. No one is entirely sure why this happens, but if being properly hydrated means you burn more fat, it's an effortless step to take!

Water is a Mood Booster.

Okay, that might not be entirely true. But water does prevent dehydration, and since some of the mental and physical effects of dehydration are fatigue, confusion, and dizziness.

Dehydration has even, in some studies, been linked to an increase in cortisol production. So, if you don't drink enough water, you're likely to be tired, stressed, and confused. Sounds like a recipe for being hangry, doesn't it?

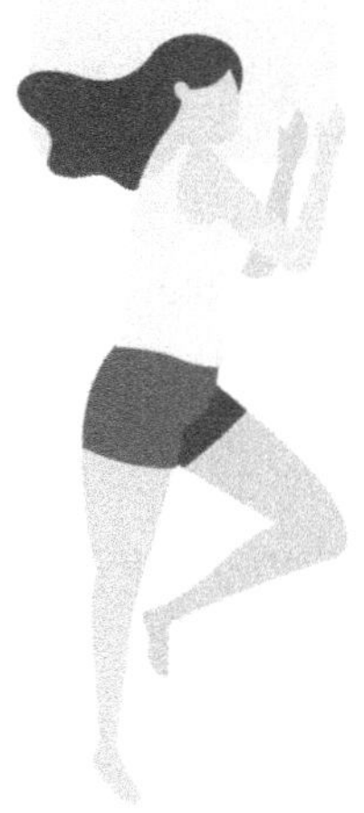

Sleep

Yes, we've said it before, but it bears repeating: not sleeping enough can make you gain weight and make it harder to lose weight.

Good sleep habits, including going to sleep at the same time every night, getting at least seven hours of sleep per night, and banishing work and entertainment devices from the bedroom, are some of the simplest things you can do to boost your metabolism. It also improves your chances of losing weight and keeping it gone.

Why wouldn't you start with all the low-hanging fruit you can and set yourself up for success!

Healthy Diet

We've already covered this in some depth, so there's not too much left to be said before we get into specifics, but it might surprise you that this is the last item in this section.

It shouldn't.

Too often, we think of weight loss and management as ONLY about what we eat. That's absolutely untrue. As you can see, there are so many other things that play a role, which might be derailing your efforts.

While it's certainly important to eat the right things, in the right proportions and at the right time, it's not the only thing you can do. So, make sure that you tackle everything else on this list while you address your eating habits, and you will be set up for success.

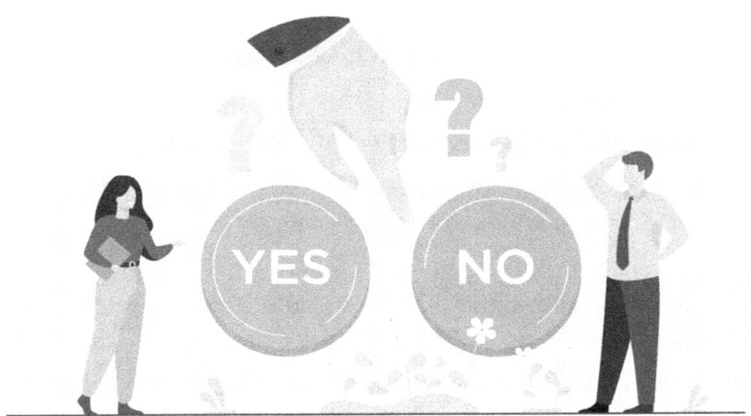

Do's and Don'ts of a Fast Metabolism

Glad you're still with me! We've covered a lot of ground so far, and you might be feeling a little bit overwhelmed about all the things you never even realized were related to your metabolism. So, we thought we'd end with a quick "do's and don'ts" cheat sheet. Here it is:

- **Don't** eat too much or too little. Both can have a detrimental effect on your metabolism!
- **Do** choose whole foods and cook them yourself whenever possible.
- **Don't** underestimate the impact of physical activity on your metabolism.
- **Do** incorporate both cardio for immediate fat burning and strength training to boost your muscle mass into your workouts.
- **Don't** overlook lifestyle factors like sleep and stress.
- **Do** take care of your general health. There are a multitude of conditions that could be slowing down your metabolism and

could be dangerous. Always speak to your doctor if you are worried.

- **Don't** forget to stay hydrated. Water is more important than you think.
- **Do** understand that changing your metabolism, losing stubborn pounds, and keeping them off is a long-term lifestyle change – not a quick fix or a miracle pill.

There's a lot more information that you could dive into on the topic of metabolism and your lifestyle. Still, even if you only focus on those few points, you'll be off to a good start! So, print them out, frame them, and put them somewhere you'll see them often.

The End of the Basics

Congratulations! We've reached the end of the background information you need to know to improve your metabolism, lose weight, and keep it gone.

All of this information may seem like a lot to take in, but it's important to know just how many factors exist to a healthy metabolism and how interconnected everything is.

If you've just been trying to lose weight and keep it off based on calorie-restrictive diets, you can probably see now why they generally don't work. You can't change only one thing and expect to succeed.

But when you know all of these other factors and take action on those, and THEN change your diet, you're setting yourself up for success.

In the next part of this book, we will look more specifically at diet and exercise and how you can make better choices. So, without further ado, let's get on with it!

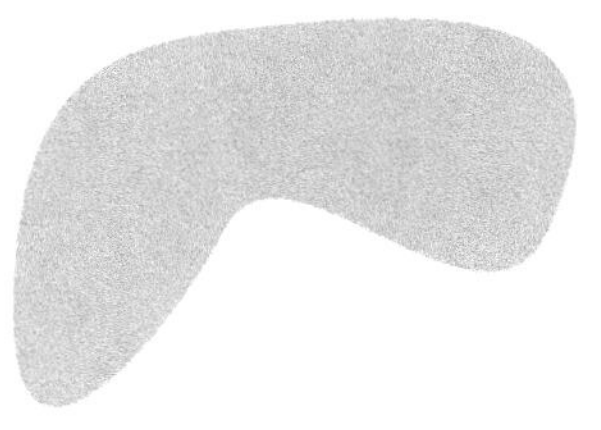

DON'T WAIT UNTIL YOU'VE REACHED YOUR GOAL TO BE PROUD OF YOURSELF. BE PROUD OF EVERY STEP YOU TAKE TOWARD REACHING THAT GOAL.

– *Unknown*

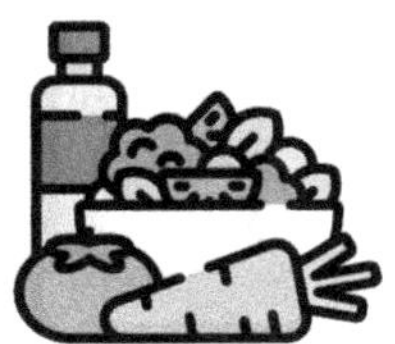

FIVE

Great Foods

For many years, the diet industry (and yes, it is an industry!) has been trying to convince us that a healthy diet is complicated. It's not.

The basics of a healthy diet are very simple: eat the right foods, in the right portions and proportions, at the right time. Don't eat too much or too little, and make sure your diet is balanced. When you say it like that, it looks so basic.

So why are we struggling?

In many ways, we're struggling because we have too many options.

Take a trip to any grocery store, and there is aisle upon aisle of options. Treats, snacks, convenience products. TV dinners for busy people. Instant meals for busy families.

There are many things to learn about healthy food, but one thing always remains true and consistent: the closer your food is to its natural state, the better it is likely to be for you. Whether fresh or frozen, vegetables, fruits, and lean meats are the basis of any healthy diet. Add some whole grains and dairy, and you have a recipe for success.

In this part of the book, we're going to take a closer look at the basics of great foods, and then we're going to teach you how to cook them.

Foods That Improve Your Metabolism

The first thing we need to say here, again, is that there are no magic bullets.

You can't make bad food choices and then just undo them by eating a few miracle foods. But there are some foods that are better for your metabolism. They include:

- Lean proteins. Whether from animal sources like meat, fish, or poultry, dairy or vegetable sources like beans, tofu, and nuts, protein helps build muscle, and muscle is good for your metabolism.
- Legumes and pulses should get a special mention here too. While they have a lot of protein that builds muscle, they are also high in fiber. This keeps you full and is low fat. So, if you want the perfect low-calorie protein option, legumes are one of the best choices.
- Foods that contain iron, selenium, and zinc, like meat, leafy greens, shellfish, or nuts. These elements help support thyroid function, and since your thyroid is a metabolic superstar, that's a good thing!
- Coffee. Believe it or not, caffeine is fantastic at kickstarting your metabolism. In fact, it can increase your metabolic rate by up to 11%! Just a few cups a day can help you burn up to 100 extra calories without changing anything else!
- Capsaicin, which is the chemical that makes chilis hot, is a

metabolism booster. Eating spicy food with capsaicin in it can help you burn up to 50 extra calories per day.

- If you don't like coffee, try tea! Tea has less caffeine than coffee, but even the smaller amount you get from tea will increase your metabolism by anything from 4% to 10%.
- Spices are also great for our metabolism and our health in general! Ginger is a known metabolism booster, as is cayenne pepper.
- Cacao (the raw form of chocolate) has been shown to prevent the absorption of some calories from fat during digestion. This may also help to speed up weight loss. But remember, we're talking about the raw version – not a slab of chocolate!
- Apple cider vinegar might also be linked to higher fat burning rates during exercise, according to some studies.
- Any foods that are lower in calories and take more effort to eat, like crunchy fruits and vegetables, are good because they encourage thermogenesis.

Again, this list isn't a list of foods that lets you eat what you like and still get results. You can't drink a cup of coffee with a burger and fries and expect to cancel out the negative effects.

But, if you're already eating a healthy, balanced diet, and you add some of these foods to the mix, you will be giving your metabolism a helping hand.

A healthy diet on its own will also help improve your metabolism. If you feed all the systems in your body the foods they need to work at their peak, everything will start working better automatically.

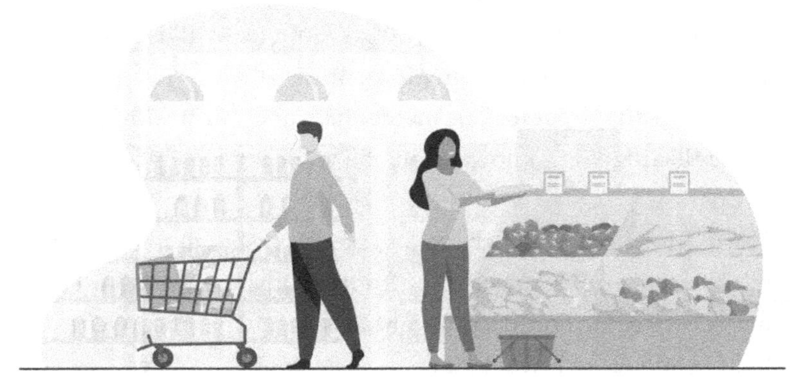

Your Shopping List

Now that you know which foods are metabolic superstars, we need to go over what you should be stocking up your fridge and pantry with to create the optimum diet.

You don't need to go to the most expensive stores or even buy organic or designer produce. Just buy the best quality you can afford and stick to the healthy choices that follow.

Protein-Rich Foods

Protein builds muscle, and muscle burns calories. So, it's only natural that we start with high protein choices. As always, choose leaner products when you can.

- Red meat, including beef, pork, and lamb, as well as ostrich (high protein with less fat than chicken!), venison, and other red meat products. Always cut off most of the visible fat on your meats because saturated fat from animal products is unhealthy.

- Poultry, including chicken, turkey, duck, and game birds. Be careful of too much duck, though, as it's a very fatty meat.
- Fish and seafood of all kinds are a great idea. Fatty fish like salmon, mackerel, and sardines also contain essential fats that are good for your health. Even canned tuna is a great choice, although it should be limited due to salt and mercury content.
- Dairy products, such as milk, yogurt, and cheese. Cottage cheese and plain yogurt are excellent choices!
- Eggs. They're one of the simplest foods and full of healthy protein. Choose omega 3 enriched eggs for an extra health boost.
- Legumes and beans, including tofu and tempeh, beans, lentils, and split peas. There are also several legume flours that can be used instead of regular flour for low-carb alternatives.
- Nuts and seeds, including pumpkin seeds, brazil nuts, peanuts, sunflower seeds, almonds, and other tree nuts and seeds.
- Vegetables can also be great protein rich foods. Some of these include spinach, asparagus, broccoli, Chinese cabbage, Brussels sprouts, cauliflower, and more.

There's been a real move towards eating more protein lately, as carbs have been cut out of our diets. This is a good choice, as long as your diet stays balanced. Still, as you can see, there's a lot of variety that falls under the protein umbrella! No need to be bored and eat just one type!

Iron, Zinc, and Selenium Rich Foods

We all know that we need vitamins to stay healthy, but there are a variety of metals and other elements that are essential to our health too. When it comes to your metabolism, iron, zinc, and selenium are some of the most important. Here are some of the foods that you can get each of them from:

Iron

- Meat, most notably red meat, but also pork and poultry.
- Seafood
- Dark green leafy vegetables
- Beans and peas
- Dried fruit and raisins
- Iron-fortified foods, like breads, pastas, and cereals

Zinc

- Oysters – gram for gram, one of the best sources of zinc
- Red meat
- Other seafood and shellfish
- Beans and other legumes
- Seeds, especially hemp seeds, pumpkin seeds, and sesame seeds
- Tree nuts and peanuts
- Dairy products
- Eggs
- Whole grains
- Potatoes (regular and sweet)
- Dark chocolate

Selenium

- Brazil nuts
- Fish and seafood
- Ham
- Pork, beef, turkey, and chicken
- Cottage cheese
- Brown rice
- Eggs
- Sunflower seeds
- Mushrooms
- Oatmeal
- Spinach
- Milk and yogurt
- Lentils
- Cashews
- Bananas

Some foods are also enriched with selenium, including pastas, breads, and whole-grain cereals.

Coffee and Tea

Caffeine has been shown to be great for boosting your metabolism, which is terrific for people who love coffee and tea.

Of course, coffee has more caffeine than tea, but if you don't love a cup of joe, you can choose black, green, or white tea – or try something exotic like chai!

. . .

Chilis and Spices

In recent years, spices have been repeatedly proven to be powerhouse health boosters. When it comes to your metabolism, it is no different. Aside from all of their other health benefits (and their ability to elevate an otherwise dull dish to something special!), spices are great for speeding up your metabolism.

Make sure your spice cupboard is well stocked with:

- Turmeric
- Cinnamon
- Cayenne pepper
- Cumin
- Ginger
- Cardamom
- Rosemary
- Black pepper
- Chilis

Legumes and Pulses

Legumes and pulses are superfoods. They're rich in protein, low in fat, and have many of the important trace vitamins and minerals we need to stay healthy. Choose any of these to add to or replace meat in your favorite dishes:

- Soybeans and soybean products like tofu and tempeh
- Peanuts
- Fresh peas and beans
- Dried beans
- Chickpeas

- Lentils
- Dried peas

Apple Cider Vinegar

Apple cider vinegar has been shown (in moderation) to help prevent weight gain and potentially aid in weight loss.

The reason for this is acetic acid, which is the acid that makes the vinegar taste sour.

It helps to support your metabolism in several important ways, including:

- Lowering blood sugar and decreasing insulin levels.
- Increasing the enzyme AMPK, which improves your ability to burn fat and blocks fat and sugar production in your liver.
- It's an appetite suppressant.

Of course, too much of any good thing is a bad idea. If you add apple cider vinegar to your diet, check with your doctor first, and always follow the moderation rule!

Seaweed

Seaweed is a superfood, which contains all sorts of vitamins and minerals, is low in fat, and adds great flavor to food.

When it comes to your metabolism, the important one is iodine.

Iodine is required by several vital organs and functions, including the thyroid, which is critical to a healthy, speedy metabolism, as we've already covered.

. . .

Coconut Oil

Coconut oil has a particular type of fat known as medium-chain triglycerides, which have been shown in some studies to help improve your metabolism.

MCTs, as they are also known, are metabolized differently from long-chain fatty acids, and they are less likely to be stored as fat.

However, while there is some evidence that coconut oil may be suitable for your metabolism, it is still a fat, and fats are calorie-dense foods. So, make sure if you do include it, you do so in moderation.

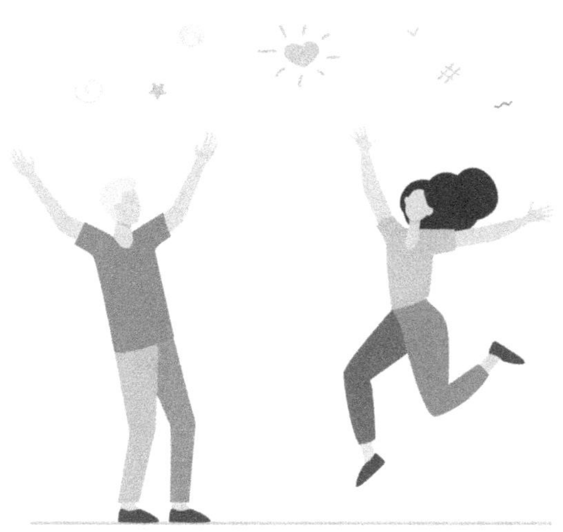

Preparing for Success

Now that you know what kinds of foods are most likely to support and improve your metabolism, the next thing you need to do is prepare for success.

If your house is stuffed to the rafters with unhealthy processed foods and snacks, you're going to be tempted to indulge, and you're going to derail any progress you make.

Either wait until you have eaten all of those things or, if you want to start right away, donate them to a local food bank or charity.

Then stock your cabinets with foods that you know are good for you. Fruits, vegetables, grains, nuts, legumes, and even a little dark chocolate are all great. Add lean meats, dairy, seafood, and eggs, and you're all set to eat for a better metabolism.

The best part? With all those foods on the menu, you don't have to eat bland, boring, tasteless food. So, let's get right into what you can eat! Easy, metabolism-friendly recipes are up next!

BALANCE IS THE KEY TO HEALTH AND SUCCESS

- Laure Carter

Recipes

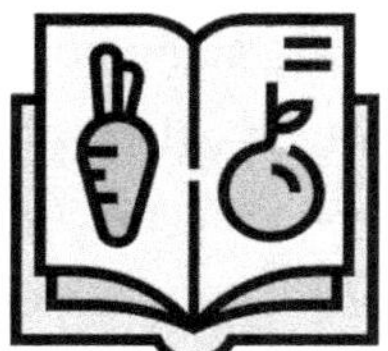

You are what you eat. That's not just a **cliché**. It's a **fact**. If you eat healthy, whole foods, you're going to be a healthier person. If you eat a lot of processed junk, you won't. It really is just that simple.

Most people want to eat healthily, but they find themselves struggling to integrate healthy eating with a busy lifestyle.

The recipes included here are as easy as possible to throw together. Still, there are also things you can do to make cooking healthy meals easier.

One is to set aside some time every week to prep vegetables and other ingredients. Another is to buy dried beans in bulk and precook them. Cooked beans freeze well in zip lock bags, and you can add them directly to many dishes without even thawing them!

Plan ahead, make sure you have all the ingredients you need for easy, healthy, metabolism-boosting recipes, and you will be much more likely to make your own healthy meals instead of reaching for bad convenience foods.

In this chapter, we're going to look at some easy, tasty, and metabolism-supportive recipes that you can make every day of the week. Eating the right food to support and speed up your metabolism doesn't have to be complicated or time-consuming, as you will see. Try these recipes as is, or substitute your favorite ingredients where you need to, to turn them into meals your whole family will enjoy or to support your eating methodologies.

Note: Some recipes may include sugar for taste, feel free to leave that out or replace this with honey. Also, all recipes can be easily be adjusted to be suitable for vegetarians or vegans. Simply substitute meat or dairy with your favorite alternatives.

Enjoy!

Breakfast

Breakfast is, as they say, the most important meal of the day, and that's especially true when it comes to your metabolism.

Eating a meal when you wake up is an important step in kickstarting your metabolism.

Skipping breakfast doesn't help you lose weight either but may make it harder for you to lose weight. So even if you don't like a huge meal first thing in the morning, try to incorporate one of these options into your routine.

EASY MEXI-EGGS

Eggs are one of the most perfect breakfast foods. They're high protein, tasty, and easy to prepare. Adding spicy salsa and a sprinkling of cheese takes them from ordinary breakfast food to something you will look forward to every day!

INGREDIENTS:

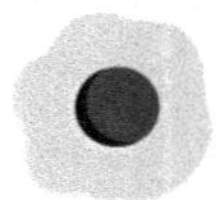
One egg per person

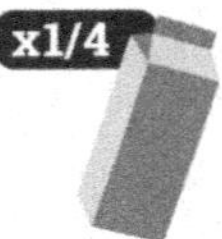
Cup of milk

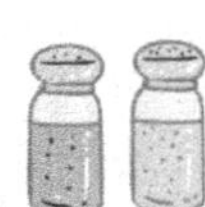
Salt and pepper to taste

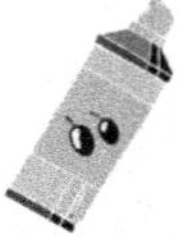
Olive oil spray

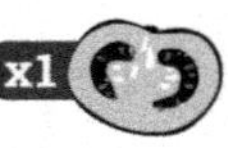
Tomato

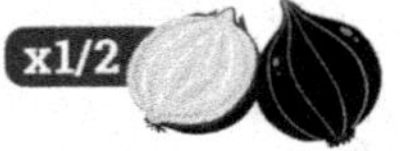
Small to medium onion

Small jalapeno

Cilantro

Lime juice

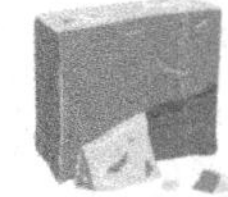
Grated cheese to serve

EASY MEXI-EGGS

METHOD

1 Finely chop the tomato, onion, jalapeno, and cilantro. Mix all the ingredients together and sprinkle with lime juice. Season with salt and pepper and set aside.

2 Mix the eggs and milk and season to taste.

3 Spray a non-stick pan with olive oil spray.

4 Scramble the eggs over medium heat until cooked through.

5 Top eggs with salsa and sprinkle a little cheese on top.

6 Microwave for 20 – 30 seconds, or just long enough to slightly melt the cheese and warm the salsa and serve.

CARAMELIZED BANANA NUT TOAST

Bananas are a metabolism booster on their own, but when you pair them with whole-grain toast and almond butter, it's a whole new level. Even better? This tasty breakfast is super easy to make and tastes soooo good.

INGREDIENTS:

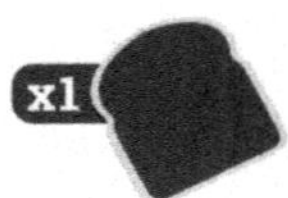

Slice of toasted whole-grain bread (choose an iron-fortified product or seed loaf to get an extra metabolism boost)

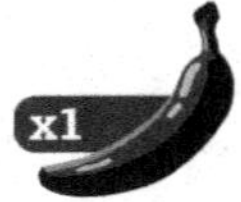

One small banana, peeled and split in half lengthwise

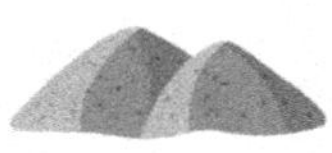

Brown sugar

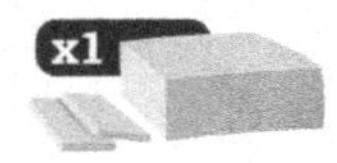

Tablespoon butter

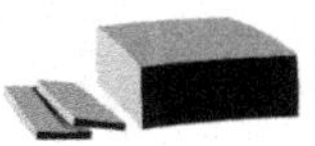

Almond butter (choose one with no added sugar or salt)

Chopped Almonds

CARAMELIZED BANANA NUT TOAST

METHOD

1 Spread toast with almond butter.

2 Heat butter in a small pan, sprinkle a little brown sugar in the pan and then add the banana, cut side down. Sprinkle a little more brown sugar on top.

3 Gently sauté the banana until caramelized and soft, then turn and repeat on the other side.

4 Serve banana on top of toast and top with chopped nuts.

BERRY YOGURT BOWL

Plain yogurt is a great metabolism-boosting choice. In fact, some studies have shown that people who eat seven or more servings of plain yogurt per week are less likely to be overweight or obese than those who don't. Berries are a great addition, and by adding some seeds, you can increase the selenium content of this easy breakfast.

INGREDIENTS:

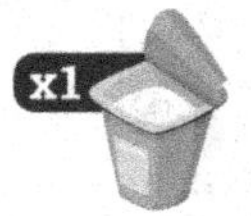

Cup of plain yogurt

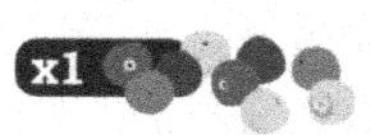

Cup of mixed berries (you can use fresh chopped berries or a frozen blend – defrosted)

Cup of mixed seeds, including sunflower seeds, chia seeds, and pumpkin seeds.

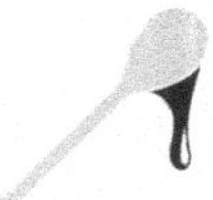

Drizzle of honey

BERRY YOGURT BOWL

METHOD

1 Place berries in a layer at the bottom of a bowl.

2 Top with plain yogurt.

3 Sprinkle with mixed seeds.

4 Drizzle honey over yogurt to taste. Plain yogurt and berries can both be a little on the tart side, so this helps to take the edge off.

MUSHROOM OMELETS

Mushrooms have a high selenium content, and eggs are packed with protein. This recipe adds cottage cheese and chives for a tasty breakfast treat that is quick and easy to make, and very tasty.

INGREDIENTS:

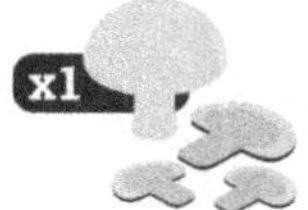

Cup of sliced mushrooms

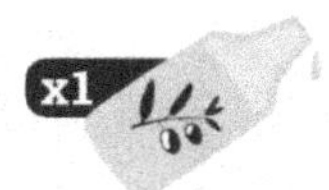

Tablespoon olive oil for sautéing

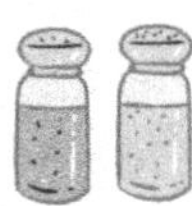

Salt and pepper to taste

Chopped chives

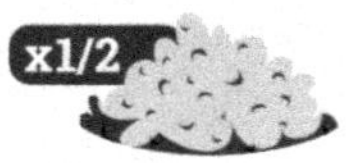

Cup cottage cheese

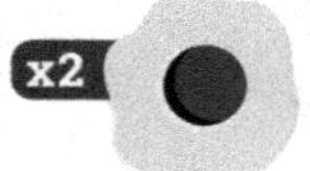

Eggs

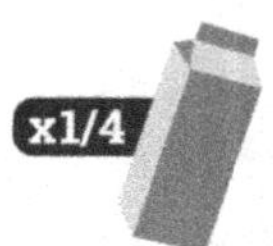

Cup of milk

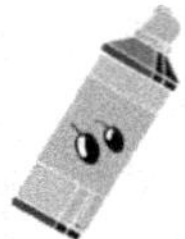

Olive oil spray

MUSHROOM OMELETS
METHOD

1 Sautee the mushrooms in a small pan with the olive oil, seasoning, and chives.

2 Mix the mushrooms with cottage cheese and keep warm.

3 Whisk eggs with milk and season.

4 Heat a non-stick pan and spray with olive oil.

5 Pour eggs in and cook over medium heat until the bottom of the omelet is set and the top is almost completely cooked.

6 If you prefer your omelet fully cooked, flip to finish cooking the other side, or you can fill and fold the omelet, slide it onto a plate and serve.

BREAKFAST HASH

Potatoes are great for metabolism, and if you don't peel them before you cook them, they've got a lot of fiber in them too. A simple and tasty breakfast hash, topped with a fried egg, is a great way to get all kinds of metabolism-friendly stuff into the first meal of the day.

INGREDIENTS:

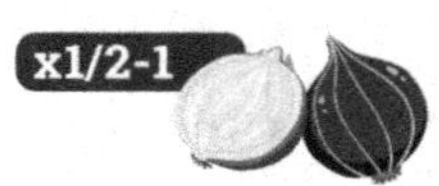

One small or half a large onion, finely chopped

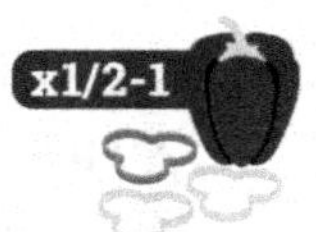

Small or half a large green or red pepper, chopped

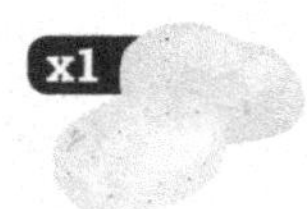

Medium to large potato, cut into 1/4 inch cubes

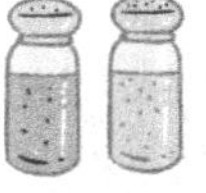

Salt and pepper to taste

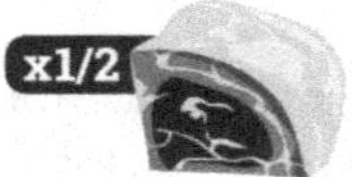

Cup of chopped ham

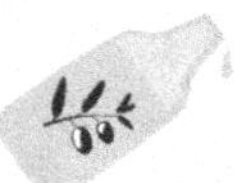

Olive oil for frying

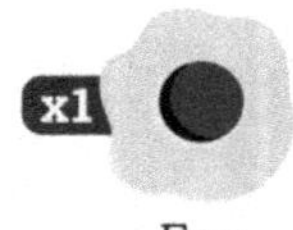

Egg

BREAKFAST HASH

METHOD

1 Parboil potatoes until they are almost cooked but still holding their shape. Drain and set aside.

2 Heat oil in a frying pan and add the onions and peppers. Stir fry until soft and onions are translucent.

3 Remove onions and peppers from the pan and set them aside.

4 Add another tablespoon of oil to the pan, and then add the reserved, par-boiled potatoes. Stir fry the potatoes over medium heat until they are golden brown, cooked through, and crispy.

5 Stir in the onions and peppers, cubed ham, and seasoning.

6 Fry egg, leaving the yolk a little runny.

7 Plate hash, top with an egg, and serve.

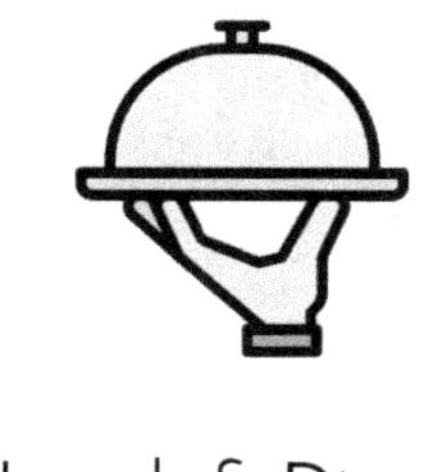

Lunch & Dinner

You might be tempted to skip meals when you're trying to lose weight. But as you've already seen, that does more harm than good. Not eating will actually cause your metabolism to slow down. In fact, if you want a healthy, speedy metabolism, the best thing you can do is to eat regular, healthy meals.

Not only is this metabolism friendly, but it will ensure that your blood sugar stays relatively constant. Big peaks and troughs in your blood sugar are a very common cause of snack cravings!

All of these meals are easy to make, use ordinary ingredients that you probably have in your pantry, and taste good too!

SALMON SALAD NIÇOISE

This classic French salad is usually made with tuna, but salmon works really well too. This is also a great way to get all sorts of metabolism-boosting superstars into your meals!

INGREDIENTS:

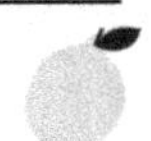
A squeeze of lemon juice

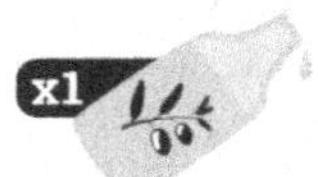
Tablespoon extra virgin olive oil

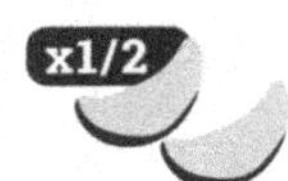
Tsp finely chopped garlic

Pinch of finely chopped fresh basil

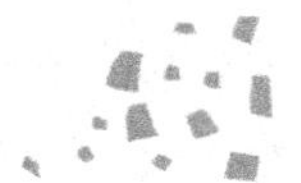
Pinch of finely chopped fresh tarragon

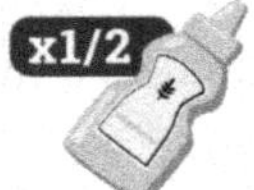
Teaspoon Dijon mustard

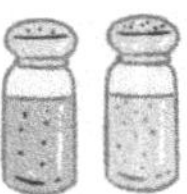
Salt and freshly ground black pepper

Poached salmon fillet

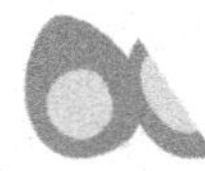
Hard-boiled egg peeled and quartered lengthwise

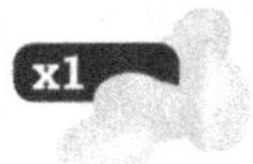
1 cup of quartered, cooked baby potatoes

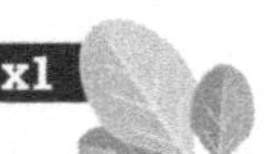
Cup of baby spinach

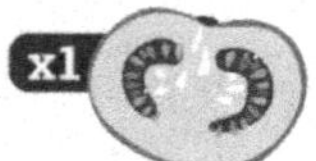
Small tomato cut into wedges.

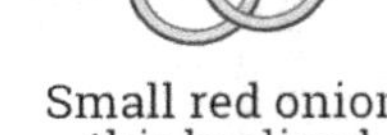
Small red onion, thinly sliced

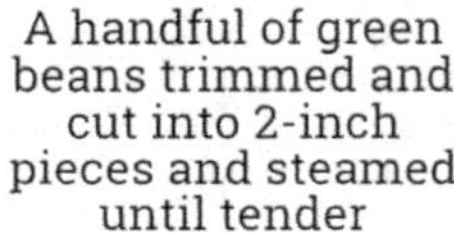
A handful of green beans trimmed and cut into 2-inch pieces and steamed until tender

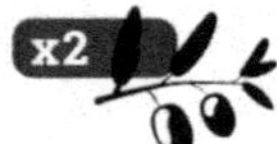
Tbsp cup niçoise olives

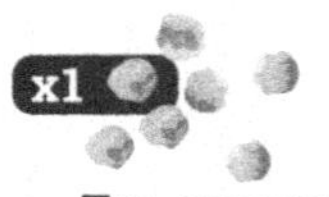
Tsp capers

SALMON SALAD NIÇOISE

METHOD

1 Mix all the ingredients up to the first measure of salt and pepper together and set aside.

2 Flake poached salad.

3 Toss spinach in 1⁄2 of the vinaigrette and arrange on a plate.

4 Top spinach with potatoes, tomatoes, onions, and green beans.

5 Scatter with olives, capers, and boiled egg.

6 Top salad with flaked salmon and drizzle with remaining vinaigrette.

HONEY SRIRACHA CHICKEN LETTUCE CUPS

Low fat protein, crunchy vegetables, sesame seeds, and a spicy sauce are an excellent choice for a tasty, metabolism-boosting lunch or dinner.

INGREDIENTS:

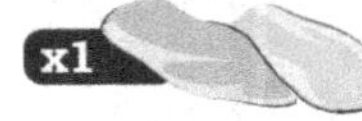

One chicken breast fillet

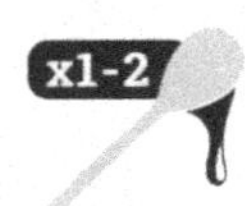

Tbsp honey

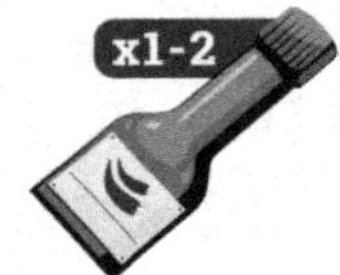

Tbsp sriracha

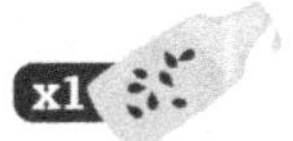

Tsp sesame oil

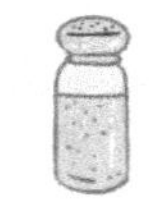

Salt to taste

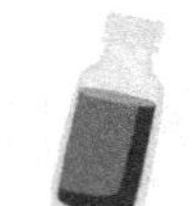

Water or chicken stock

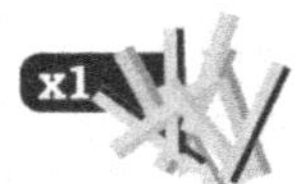

Small carrot cut into matchsticks

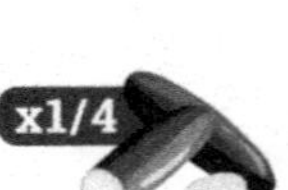

Cucumber, cut into matchsticks

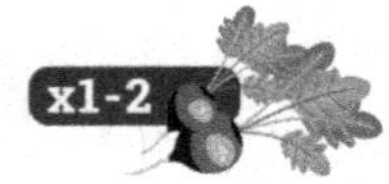

Radishes cut into matchsticks

Small, soft-leaved lettuce (butter, bib, or even romaine work well)

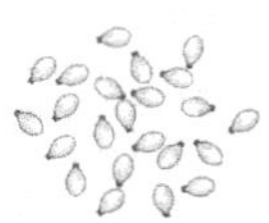

Sesame seeds for serving

HONEY SRIRACHA CHICKEN LETTUCE CUPS

METHOD

1 Heat sesame oil in a pan, add the chicken, season with salt, and fry lightly on each side, until starting to brown.

2 Add 1 to 2 cups of water or chicken stock to the pan, cover with the lid and continue to steam, occasionally turning until chicken is cooked through.

3 Just before the water is all gone, add the honey and sriracha to the pan, and use two forks to shred the chicken. If the pan is too dry for the sauce to coat the chicken, add a little more.

4 Allow chicken to cool slightly, then toss with the matchstick vegetables.

5 Place rinsed lettuce leaves on a plate.

6 Fill each leaf with some of the vegetable and chicken mixture.

7 Sprinkle with sesame seeds and serve.

PEA AND HAM SOUP

Split peas, like all pulses, are perfect for your metabolism, as are ham and potatoes. This soup is easy to make, tasty, and freezes well – so you can keep the leftovers for a day you don't feel like cooking! If you love bread with your soup, serve with a whole-grain or seed bread for extra metabolism boost and fiber.

INGREDIENTS:

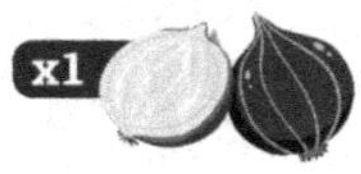

Small onion, chopped

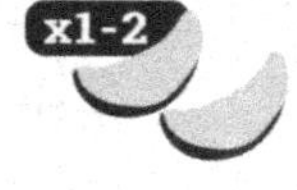

Cloves of garlic, chopped

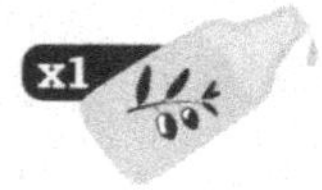

Olive oil

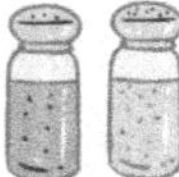

Salt and pepper, to taste

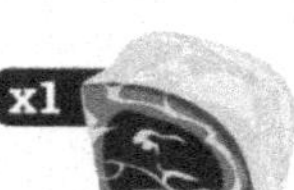

Cup of ham, cubed

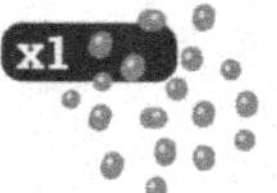

Package of split peas

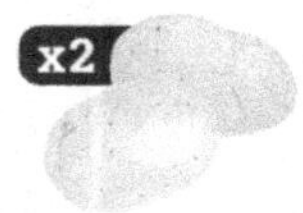

Small potatoes cut into 1/2 inch cubes

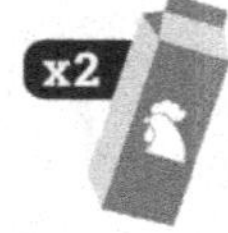

Cartons of chicken stock

PEA AND HAM SOUP

METHOD

1 Heat oil in a heavy-based soup pot.

2 Add onion and salt and sauté until softened.

3 Add garlic and ham and stir fry until fragrant but be careful – garlic burns fast!

4 Pour chicken stock into the pot.

5 Add the split peas and potatoes.

6 Bring to the boil, then turn down to a simmer and simmer, covered, stirring occasionally, for 2 to 3 hours or until the peas are softened.

7 Check and adjust the seasoning and serve.

STEAK TACOS

Lean red meat is a great source of protein, and these tacos are packed full of tasty vegetables as well. You can use hard or soft tacos or tortillas for this, depending on what you like. When it's thinly sliced, one steak goes a long way, so there's a good chance you will get two meals out of one!

INGREDIENTS:

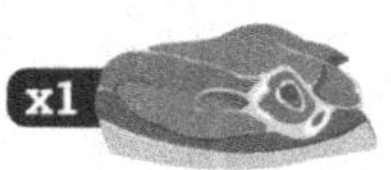
Medium-sized steak

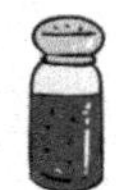
Taco seasoning

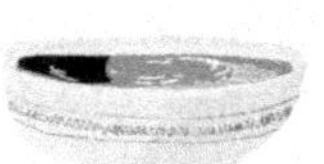
Worcestershire sauce

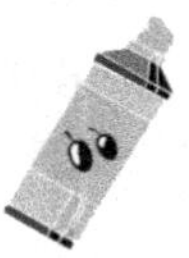
Olive oil spray

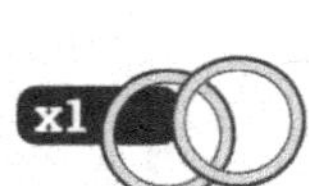
Thinly sliced red onion

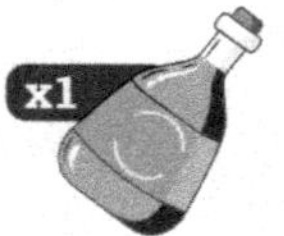
Cup red wine vinegar

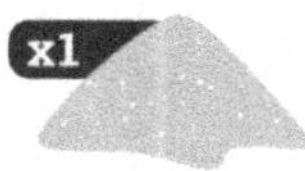
Tsp sugar

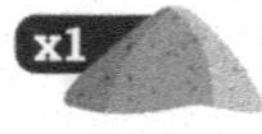
Tsp chili flakes

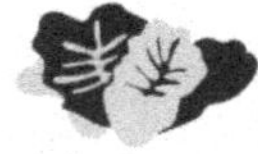
Shredded lettuce

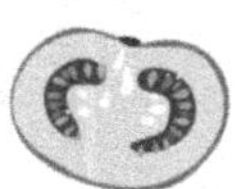
Diced tomatoes

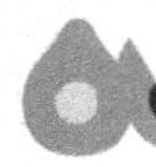
Diced avocado

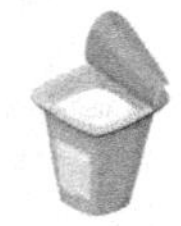
Plain yogurt

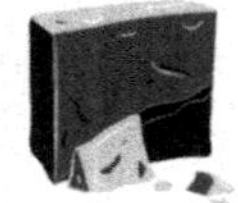
A sprinkling of cheddar cheese

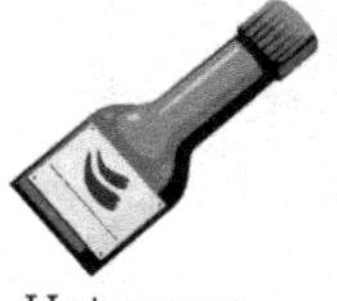
Hot sauce (optional)

Corn or flour tortillas or taco shells

STEAK TACOS

METHOD

1 Rub steak with Worcestershire sauce, and dip both sides in taco seasoning.

2 Heat oil in a heavy (preferably cast iron) pan.

3 Place steak in the pan to sear.

4 In a glass bowl, mix the onions, vinegar, sugar, and chili flakes. Microwave on high for a minute, stir, and allow the onions to sit in the vinegar mixture.

5 When the steak releases easily and is seared on the first side, turn it over and repeat on the other side.

6 When the steak is done to your liking, remove it from the pan and set aside to rest.

7 Mix the tomatoes and the avocado.

8 To assemble the tacos, place a little lettuce on each taco, and top with the tomato and avocado mixture.

9 Thinly slice the steak, about 5mm or 1/4 inch thick.

10 Place the hot steak on the vegetables, sprinkle with cheese, and then top with a spoon of plain yogurt and some hot sauce.

CHICKEN SATAY SALAD

Chicken satay is a great dish, but it's a bit fussy to make every day. Who has time to thread chicken onto skewers anyway? This salad combines all the best things about chicken satay with a mixture of brown rice, vegetables, and fruit.

INGREDIENTS:

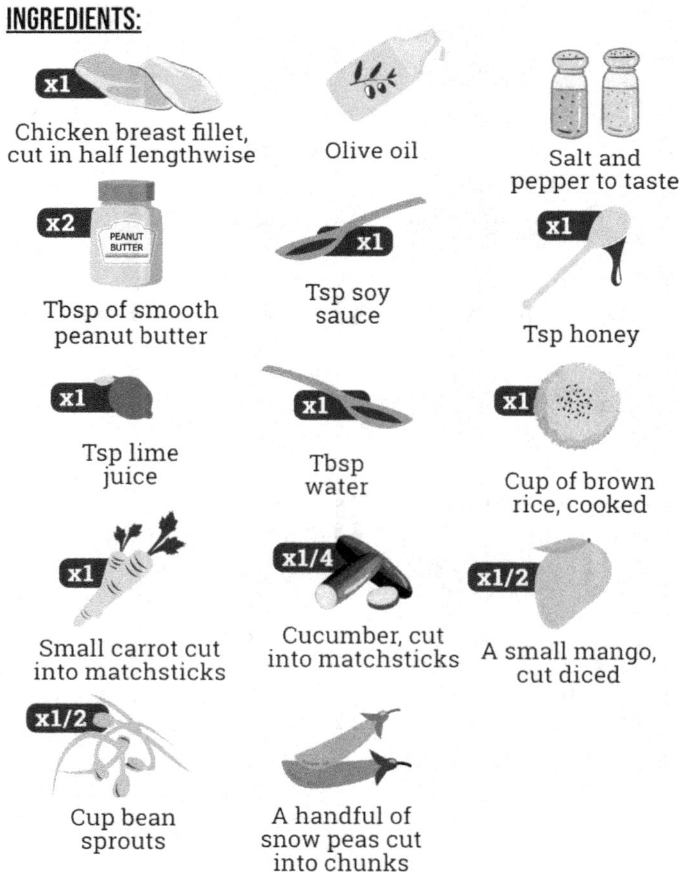

x1 Chicken breast fillet, cut in half lengthwise

Olive oil

Salt and pepper to taste

x2 Tbsp of smooth peanut butter

x1 Tsp soy sauce

x1 Tsp honey

x1 Tsp lime juice

x1 Tbsp water

x1 Cup of brown rice, cooked

x1 Small carrot cut into matchsticks

x1/4 Cucumber, cut into matchsticks

x1/2 A small mango, cut diced

x1/2 Cup bean sprouts

A handful of snow peas cut into chunks

CHICKEN SATAY SALAD

METHOD

1 Heat oil in a pan.

2 Season the chicken and cook over medium heat until slightly golden on the outside and cooked through.

3 Mix the peanut butter, soy sauce, honey, lime juice, and water to form a smooth dressing. It should be a pourable consistency, but not too thin.

4 Mix the rice, vegetables, mango, and bean sprouts together.

5 Slice the chicken into thin strips.

6 Serve chicken over rice salad, drizzled with peanut sauce.

KOREAN PORK BOWLS

Korean food is made of simple ingredients, but it's super tasty, thanks to the many spices used in their dishes. This pork bowl combines thinly sliced, highly spiced pork with brown rice and some vegetables to tone down the heat! This makes enough pork for two, or you can save some for later!

INGREDIENTS:

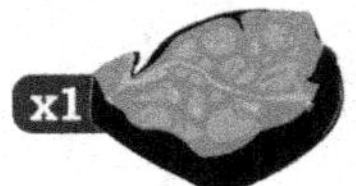
One small pork fillet very thinly sliced across the grain.

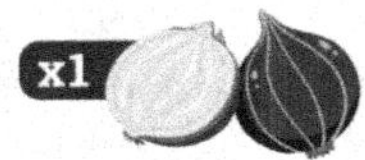
Small onion very thinly sliced

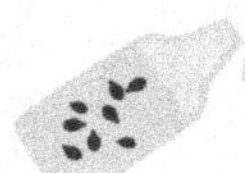
Sesame oil

Tablespoons of apple sauce

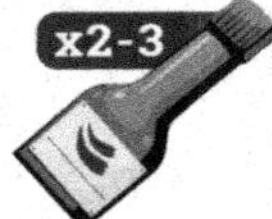
tablespoons of gochujang (Korean chili paste) or sriracha.

Tbsp soy sauce

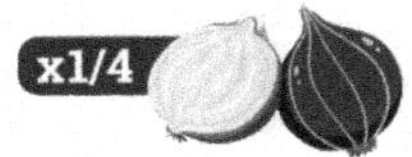
Small onion

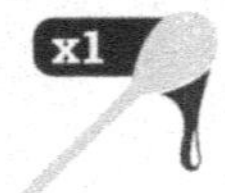
Tbsp honey

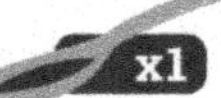
Tsp mirin

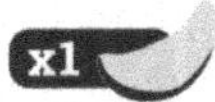
Clove of garlic, crushed

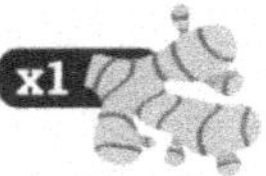
Tsp minced ginger

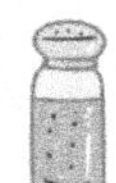
A pinch of black pepper

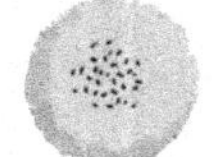
Cooked brown rice to serve

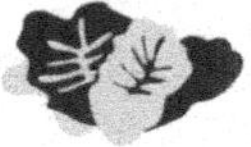
Shredded lettuce to serve

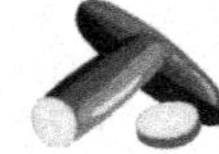
Sliced cucumber to serve

Spring onions to garnish

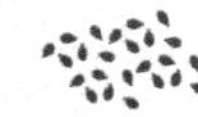
Sesame seeds to garnish

KOREAN PORK BOWLS

METHOD

1 Blend all of the ingredients from the apple sauce to the black pepper together and use it to marinate the pork for a few minutes.

2 Heat the sesame oil in a wok or heavy frying pan.

3 Stir fry pork with the onions and marinade until cooked through and onion are softened.

4 Spoon rice into bowls. Top with pork mixture and serve with lettuce and cucumber on the side.

5 Sprinkle with sesame seeds and green onion and serve.

VEGETARIAN TACO SOUP

Taco soup is a very satisfying meal, and when you use beans, you won't even miss the meat. If you can't live without a bit of meat in your meal, you can add some shredded chicken or pork to this dish if you prefer.

INGREDIENTS:

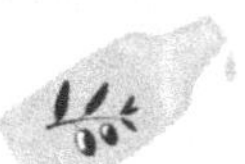
Olive oil

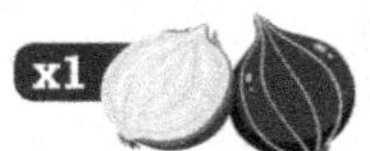
Small onion, chopped

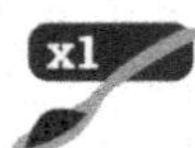
Tablespoon of taco seasoning

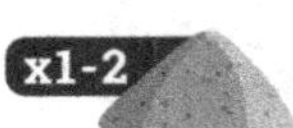
Tsp chili flakes

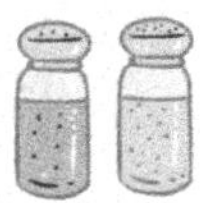
Salt and pepper to taste

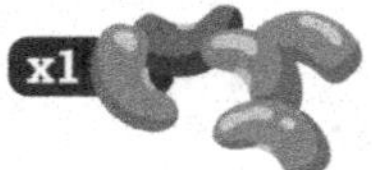
Can of black beans drained and rinsed

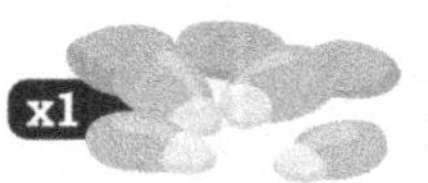
Can of corn rinsed and drained

Small green pepper, cubed

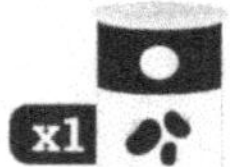
Large can of tomatoes, pureed

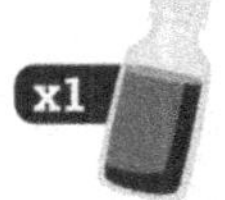
Carton of vegetable or chicken stock

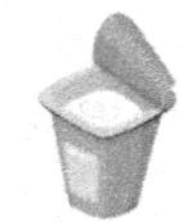
Plain yogurt, to serve

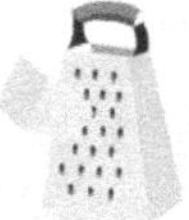
Shredded cheese to serve

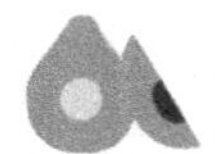
Cubed avocado to serve

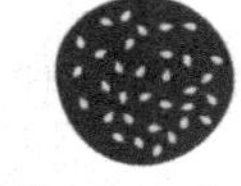
Whole-wheat tortillas, to serve (optional)

VEGETARIAN TACO SOUP

METHOD

1 Heat about a tablespoon of olive oil in a heavy-bottomed saucepan or Dutch oven.

2 Add onion, taco seasoning, chili flakes, and salt and pepper, and cook until the onion begins to soften. If the mixture becomes too dry, you can add a little water to prevent it from burning.

3 When the onions are soft, add all the vegetables, including the canned tomatoes and the stock.

4 Cover and simmer for about 45 minutes, or until all the vegetables are soft and the liquid has reduced a little.

5 Taste the soup and adjust the seasoning.

6 Serve soup with plain yogurt, cheese, cubed avocado, and tortillas for dipping.

7 You can also use the tortillas and cheese to make quesadillas, which are very nice dipped in this spicy soup!

SCOTCH EGGS

Scotch eggs are a delicious way to get a lot of healthy protein for lunch or dinner. They're easy to make once you get the hang of it, and you can serve them with any sort of salad you like. This recipe is for two eggs, but you can easily increase the quantities for more people.

INGREDIENTS:

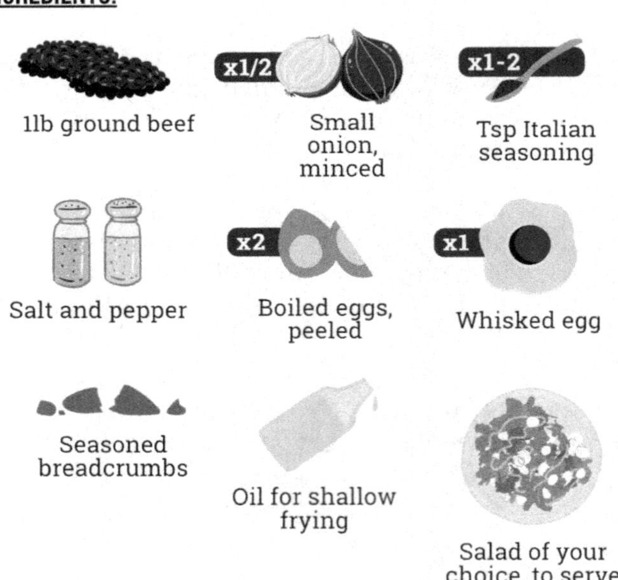

1lb ground beef

Small onion, minced

Tsp Italian seasoning

Salt and pepper

Boiled eggs, peeled

Whisked egg

Seasoned breadcrumbs

Oil for shallow frying

Salad of your choice, to serve

SCOTCH EGGS

METHOD

1 Mix the beef, onion, and seasoning together very well.

2 Heat a thin layer of oil in a frying pan.

3 Divide the meat mixture into two.

4 Place one hard-boiled egg in the center of each part of the meat mixture and press it around the egg. There should be no gaps in the meat layer, and it should be tightly pressed around the meat.

5 Dip the meatballs into the whisked egg, rolling to cover all sides.

6 Roll the dipped meatballs in breadcrumbs.

7 Place meatballs in the oil, and fry over medium heat, frequently turning, on all sides, until the breadcrumbs are golden and the meat is cooked through.

8 Serve with a salad and condiments of your choice.

TURKEY MEATLOAF BITES

Turkey is a high protein, low-fat meat option that works well in all kinds of dishes. In this one, make easy portion-sized servings of meatloaf that you can serve with salad and mashed potatoes or steamed vegetables. These meatloaf bites freeze well too, so you have easy meals on hand.

INGREDIENTS:

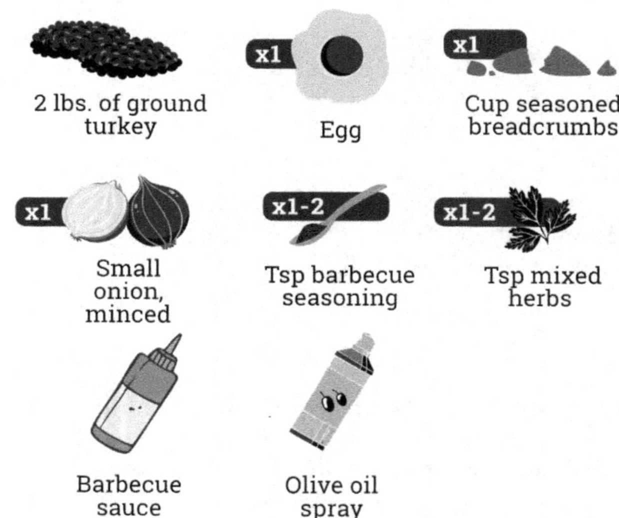

TURKEY MEATLOAF BITES

METHOD

1 Preheat oven to 350F.

2 Mix all ingredients except barbecue sauce and oil together well.

3 Lightly grease a muffin pan.

4 Press mixture into muffin pan.

5 Brush tops of meat mixture with barbecue sauce.

6 Bake until meat is cooked, and the edges of meatloaf bites are brown and slightly crisp.

EASY SALMON AND SPINACH PASTA BAKE

This pasta bake recipe tastes like comfort food, but it's full of metabolism-boosting ingredients. Using whole-wheat pasta increases the fiber content too, so it's even better for you!

INGREDIENTS:

Salmon fillets, poached, skin removed, and flaked

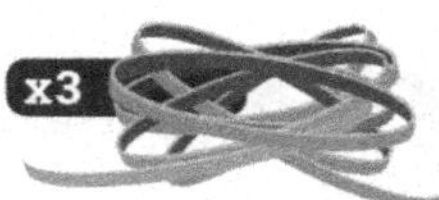

Cups of cooked whole grain pasta

Bag of chopped spinach, defrosted

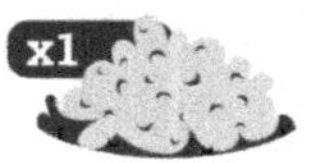

One container of cottage cheese (if you like, you can use a flavored cottage cheese, like one with chives or herbs added)

Cup of plain yogurt

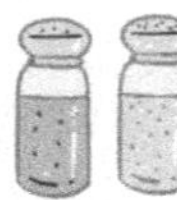

Salt and pepper to taste

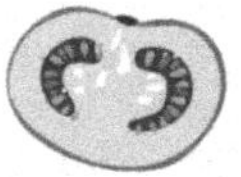

Sliced tomatoes

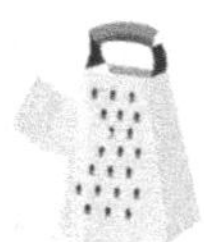

Grated cheese

EASY SALMON AND SPINACH PASTA BAKE

1 Preheat oven to 350F.

2 Mix the fish, pasta, spinach, cottage cheese, and yogurt and season to taste.

3 Spoon mixture into a prepared oven dish and smooth the top of the pasta.

4 Add a layer of sliced tomatoes and sprinkle with cheese.

5 Bake until the cheese is melted and beginning to brown.

LOADED BAKED SWEET POTATOES

Sweet potatoes can be pretty big. If you get some that are, you can serve one-half per person. This dish is somewhere between a potato skin and a twice-baked potato, and even with a sprinkling of crumbled bacon, it's full of things that are good for you!

INGREDIENTS:

One small or 1/2 large, sweet potato, baked and cut in half lengthwise

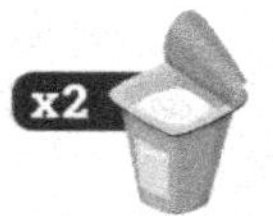

Tbsp plain yogurt

Chopped green onions

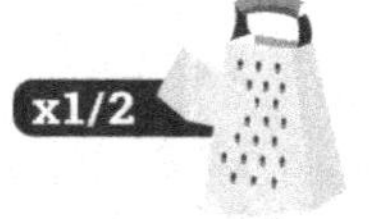

Cup grated cheese

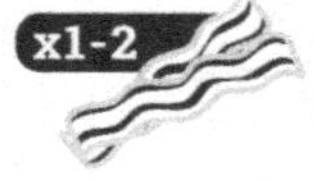

Crispy bacon strips, drained and crumbled

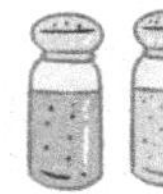

Salt and pepper to taste

LOADED BAKED SWEET POTATOES

METHOD

1 Preheat oven to 350F.

2 Scoop the center of the sweet potato into a bowl, leaving at least half an inch of flesh around the edges.

3 Mash the scooped-out sweet potato, and mix with yogurt, bacon, green onions, and half the cheese. Season to taste.

4 Spoon the mixture back into the sweet potato shells, and top with remaining cheese.

5 Bake sweet potatoes in the oven until warm, and the cheese is melted and bubbling.

VEGETARIAN BIRYANI

Biryani is an Indian rice dish that combines various spices with vegetables and meat (or just vegetables in this case), lentils, rice, potatoes, and boiled eggs. With all the spices, lentils, rice, and veggies in this dish, it's a metabolism-boosting powerhouse.

INGREDIENTS:

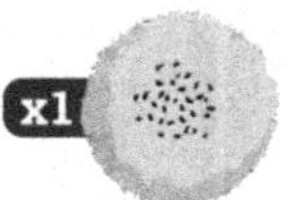
Cup basmati rice soaked in water for half an hour

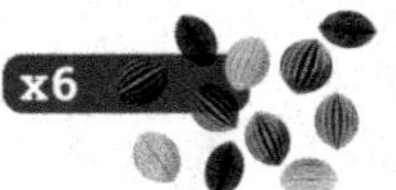
Cardamom pods

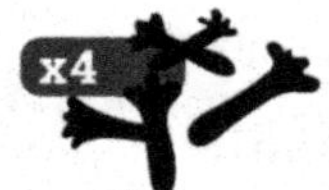
Cloves

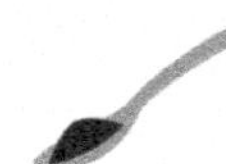
Teaspoon salt

Pinch of saffron or 1/2 tsp turmeric

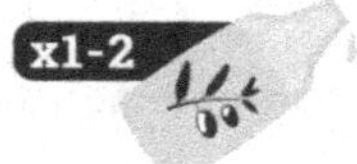
Tablespoons ghee or olive oil

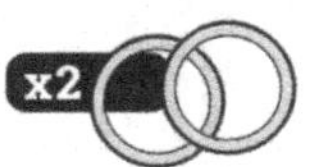
Medium red onions thinly sliced

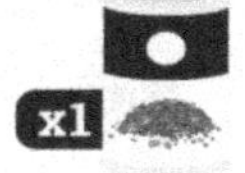
One can of lentils drained and rinsed

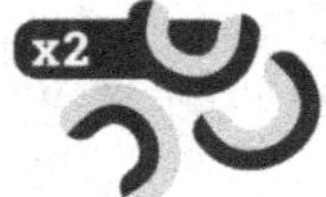
Tablespoons chopped cashews

Cup yogurt

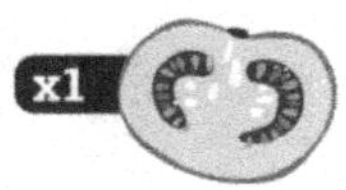
Small tomato

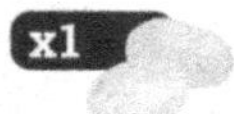
Small potato cubed

Cup cauliflower florets

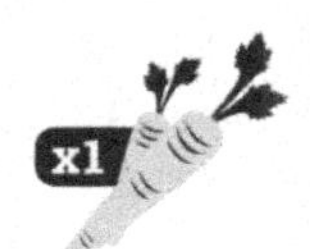
Medium carrot cut into chunks

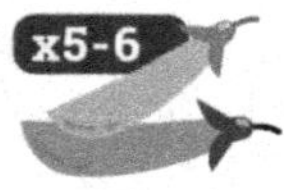
Green beans cut into chunks

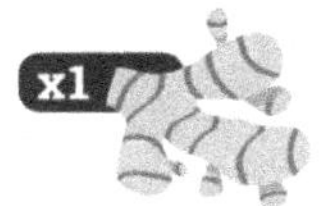

1 Inch minced ginger

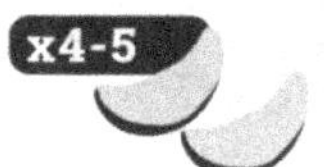

Large, crushed garlic cloves

Green chilies minced

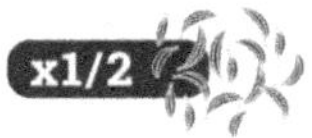

Teaspoon cumin seeds

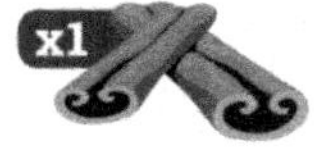

1-Inch cinnamon stick

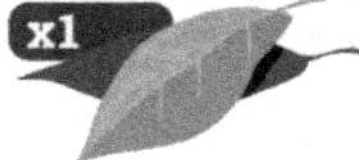

Bay leaf

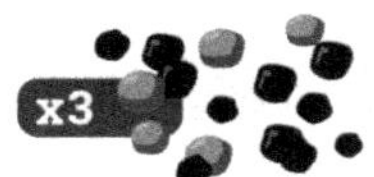

Whole black peppercorns

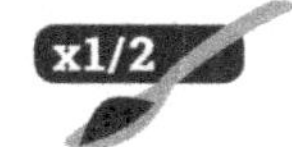

Teaspoon biryani masala

Teaspoon chili powder

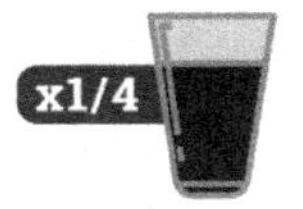

Cup of water

Tablespoons chopped cilantro

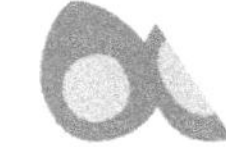

Hard-boiled eggs peeled and halved to serve

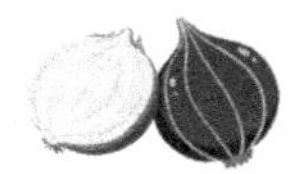

Crispy onions to serve

VEGETARIAN BIRYANI

METHOD

1 Drain rice.

2 Heat ghee in a saucepan and fry all spices and onion up to lentils until fragrant and softening.

3 Add rice and two cups of water to the pot.

4 Cook until rice is tender.

5 Stir in lentils and cashews.

6 Blend yogurt with tomato and stir in all vegetables and remaining spices.

7 Heat ghee in another saucepan and add vegetable and spice mixture to pot. Stir fry over medium heat. Add a small amount of water when the pan becomes too dry. The yogurt, tomato, and spices will become a sauce as you stir, and the vegetables will soften.

8 Serve the vegetable sauce over the rice and lentil mixture, topped with crispy onions, halved eggs, and chopped cilantro.

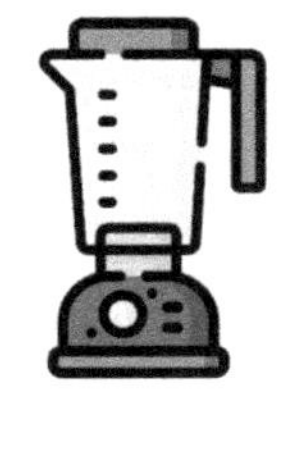

Shakes

When you can't find the time to eat a healthy breakfast or lunch, a shake made with the right kind of ingredients can make all the difference. Each of these shakes includes a variety of metabolism-boosting, healthy ingredients, so they taste great and are good for you too!

All you need to make these tasty shakes and smoothies is a blender and a few minutes to spare.

FROZEN BANANA SHAKE

Frozen bananas are a popular treat at carnivals. These shakes taste just like them but are much healthier and full of metabolism- boosting ingredients!

INGREDIENTS:

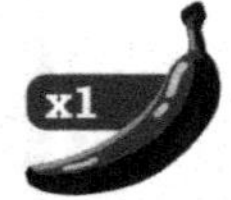

Medium banana, frozen

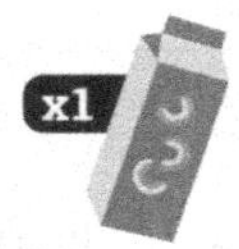

Cup of almond or cashew milk, unsweetened

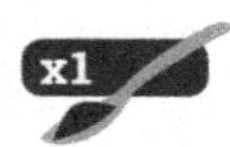

Tbsp cocoa powder

Optional

1 tsp stevia (or sugar if you prefer)

GOOD FOR YOU PINA COLADA

We all know the classic cocktail, but the ingredients in a pina colada can also be a healthy, metabolism-boosting treat!

INGREDIENTS:

Cup frozen pineapple

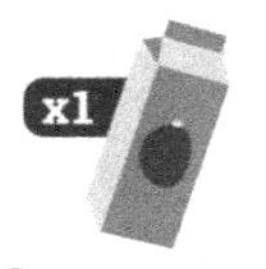

Cup coconut milk

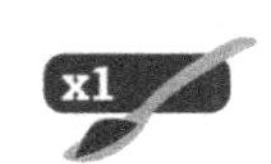

Tsp cinnamon

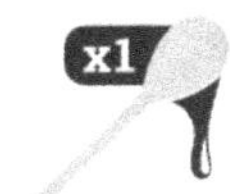

Tbsp honey

GREEN MATCHA SHAKE

Matcha has changed a lot of things. It's in all sorts of desserts and drinks. Because it's green tea powder, it's full of antioxidants and has a little caffeine kick to help kick start your metabolism.

INGREDIENTS:

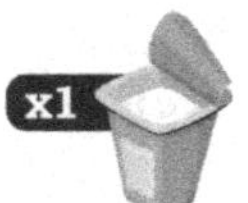

Cup plain yogurt

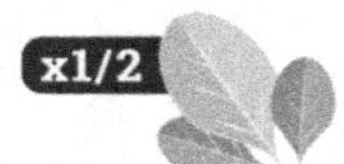

Cup packed baby spinach leaves

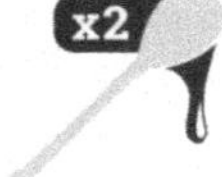

Tsp honey

A few mint leaves

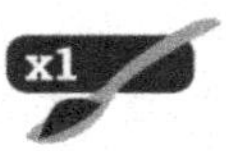

Tsp matcha powder

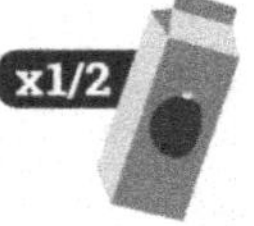

Cup coconut milk to thin

PUMPKIN PIE SMOOTHIE

There's a reason why, at a certain time of year, everything gets pumpkin spice added to it! It's delicious! This smoothie tastes like pumpkin pie, but it's good for you!

INGREDIENTS:

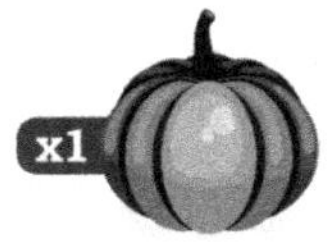

Cup of cooked
pumpkin chunks

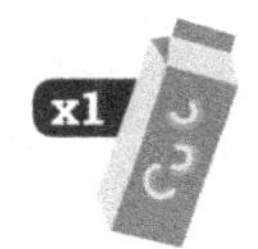

Cup of almond
or cashew milk,
unsweetened

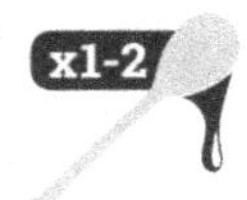

Teaspoons of
maple syrup to
sweeten

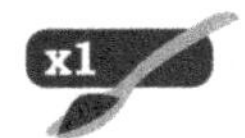

Tsp pumpkin
spice

MIXED BERRY SMOOTHIE

Berries are a fantastic food. They're low in fat, don't cause your blood sugar to spike as much as other fruits, are packed with fiber, and taste great. Plus, they make a great smoothie ingredient!

INGREDIENTS:

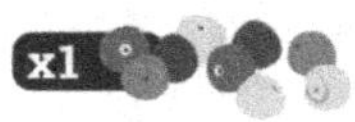 **x1** Cup frozen berries (you can use just one, like strawberry or blue- berry, or buy a mix)

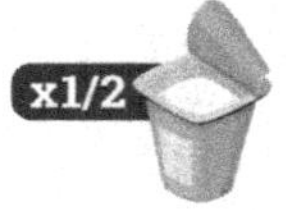 **x1/2** Cup plain yogurt

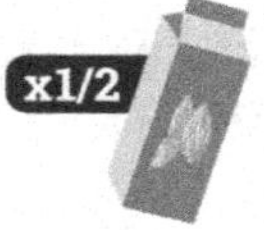 **x1/2** Cup almond milk

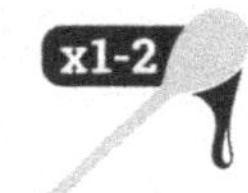 **x1-2** Teaspoons of honey

 **x1/2** Tsp cinnamon

Snacks

Some people say snack like it's a dirty word. But the truth is that snacks aren't bad for you. In fact, having a snack between meals can do your metabolism a world of good.

The trick is to choose the right kind of snack.

These snacks are all made from simple, healthy ingredients that are proven to boost your metabolism, so you can have them guilt-free!

SWEET AND SPICY NUTS AND SEEDS

There's nothing simpler than this recipe, and it makes a great snack mix that you can keep in a sealed jar. If you plan to keep it for a while, you might want to store it in the fridge, as nuts and seeds can go rancid if left too long at room temperature. Enjoy a handful at a time, but remember that while nuts and seeds are healthy, they do also have a high-fat content.

INGREDIENTS:

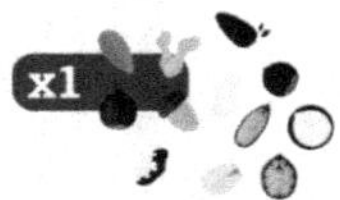

x1 Cup mixed nuts (brazil nuts, almonds, cashews, and peanuts, or any combination of them that you like)

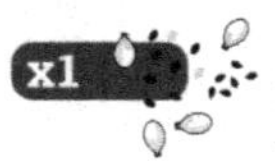

x1 Cup mixed seeds (sunflower seeds, pumpkin seeds)

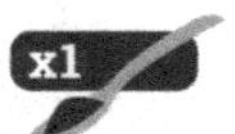

x1 Tsp chipotle chili powder

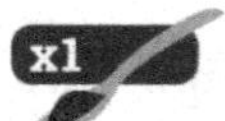

x1 Tsp brown sugar

Optional

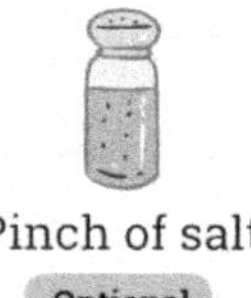

Pinch of salt

Optional

SWEET AND SPICY NUTS AND SEEDS

METHOD

1 Heat a pan.

2 Add the nuts and seeds to the pan over a low to medium heat.

3 Sprinkle the chili powder, salt, and sugar over the nuts, and toss to coat and lightly toast.

4 Remove from the heat, cool, and store.

TUNA MAYO CUCUMBER SNACKS

Tuna is a fatty fish that's a great metabolism booster. Mixed with a bit of mayo and served on slices of cucumber, they're the easiest thing in the world when you feel like having a little snack. A whole can of tuna will make a lot of tuna mayo, so you can keep this in the fridge and enjoy this snack a few times!

INGREDIENTS:

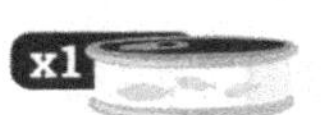

Can light meat tuna in brine, drained

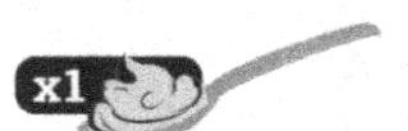

Tbsp mayonnaise

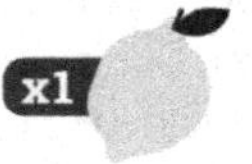

Squeeze of lemon

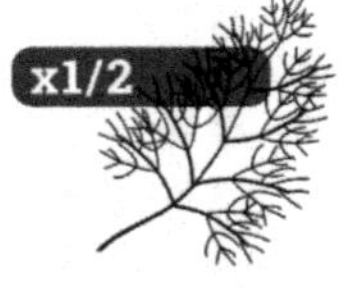

Tsp dried dill

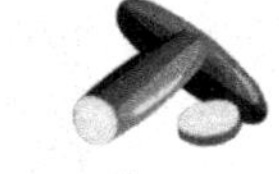

Cucumber rounds to serve

TUNA MAYO CUCUMBER SNACKS

METHOD

1 Mix the tuna with the mayonnaise, lemon, and dill.

2 Spoon a small amount of the mixture on cucumber rounds and enjoy!

HUMMUS

Hummus is a fantastic snack that is easy to make and can be enjoyed in many different ways. You can eat it with crackers, vegetables, or as a spread on toast.

INGREDIENTS:

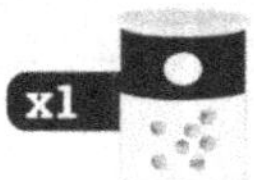

x1 Can chickpeas

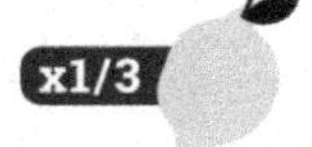

x1/3 Cup lemon juice

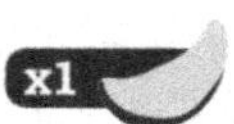

x1 Clove of garlic, crushed

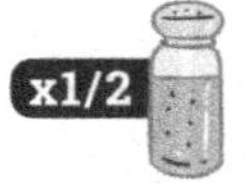
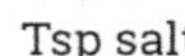

x1/2 Tsp salt

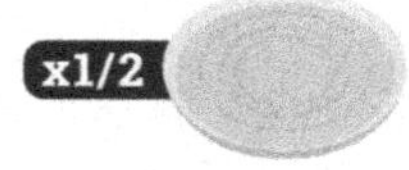

x1/2 Cup tahini

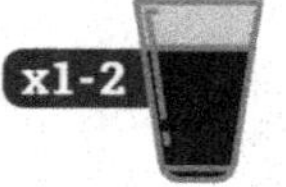

x1-2 Tbsp water

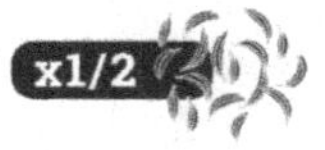

x1/2 Tsp ground cumin

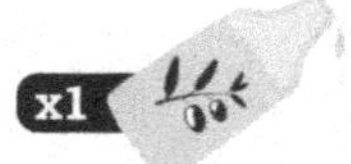

x1 Tbsp olive oil

HUMMUS

1 Blend all the ingredients together until smooth.

2 Add more water as needed to get the consistency you prefer.

3 Adjust seasoning as needed.

4 You can add many different kinds of ingredients to hummus to change the flavor. Try spicy North African harissa, or use roasted red peppers, cilantro, and parsley, or roasted garlic.

SWEET POTATO CHIPS

Chips are bad. At least, the ones you buy at the grocery store usually are. They've got too much oil, too much salt, and too many flavorings. But chips aren't all bad. These sweet potato chips are actually good for you! Enjoy with hummus or on their own.

INGREDIENTS:

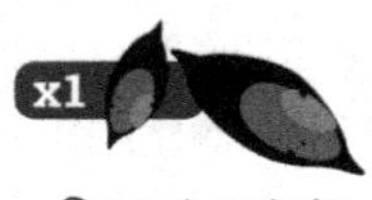

Sweet potato

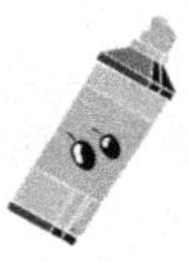

Olive oil spray

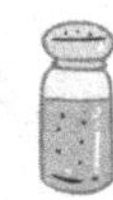

Sea salt

SWEET POTATO CHIPS

METHOD

1 Preheat your oven to 350F.

2 Use a mandolin or potato peeler to cut sweet potatoes into very thin slices.

3 Lightly grease a baking sheet and place sweet potato slices in a single layer. Spray top with a light coating of oil.

4 Bake chips in the oven until crisp.

5 Remove and toss with seas salt.

6 Keep these chips in an airtight container when totally cooled to keep them crisp. You can also use beets, carrots, and other root vegetables to make these kinds of chips.

Vegetables or Fruit and Nut Butters

The last snack idea on this list isn't a recipe. It's a pairing.

A variety of fruits and vegetables, including celery, apples, baby carrots, and others, can all be paired with nut butters. Whether you go for the classic peanut or choose almond or cashew.

Don't Starve Yourself

As you can see from these recipes, eating to support your metabolism is not about starving yourself.

You should aim to eat three meals and two or three snacks, spread out over the course of the day, to help your metabolism work at its best.

As you know from previous chapters, your metabolism is influenced by many other things, like insulin and sugar levels, fatigue, and more. By keeping your blood sugar stable and making good food choices, you will find that it's easier to get to and maintain a healthy weight, without starving yourself.

But, as important as food is, it's not everything. So, it's time to move on to all the other things you can do to keep your metabolism working at its peak and help lose (and keep off) those extra pounds.

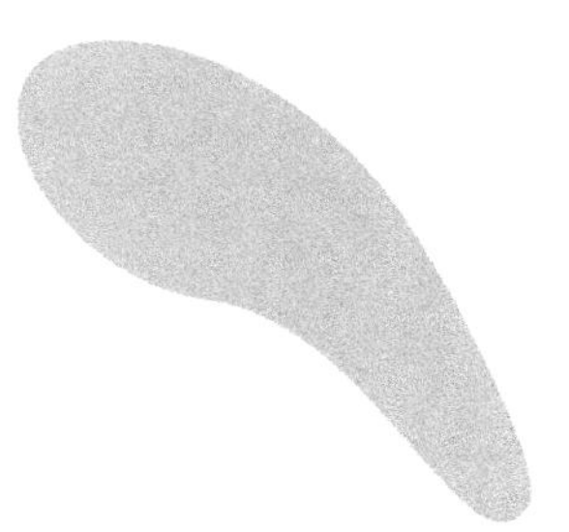

I DON'T THINK I'LL EVER
GROW OLD AND SAY,
"WHAT WAS I THINKING
EATING ALL THOSE FRUITS
AND VEGETABLES?

– Nancy S. Mure

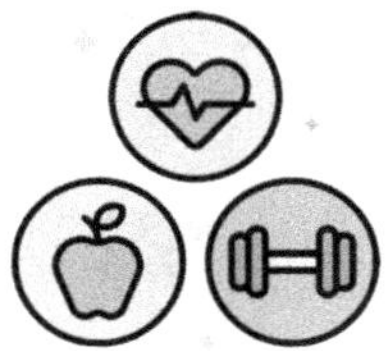

SIX

Lifestyle & Maintenance

Until you read this book, you probably also thought that losing weight and keeping it off was just a matter of cutting calories. That's a small part of it, but as you can see now, there's a whole lot more to it than that.

In this chapter, we're going to take a closer look at the lifestyle factors that affect your metabolism and how you can make positive changes to take control of them too.

If you can manage what you eat, when you eat, how much exercise you do, and all the lifestyle factors in this chapter, you will have the perfect recipe for lasting health. So, let's get to it.

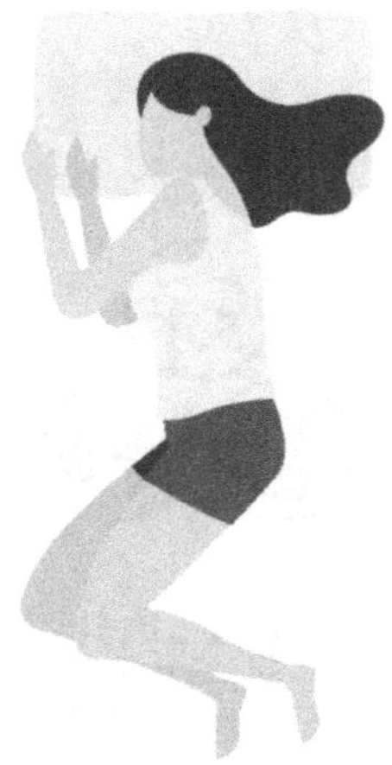

Sleep, Glorious Sleep

We've already told you that sleep is critical to supporting your metabolism, losing weight, getting fitter, and keeping in shape for the long haul.

But if you spend your nights staring at the ceiling instead of snoozing, that's not particularly helpful. So here are some practical steps you can take to sleep better.

Rule Out Medical Conditions

Sometimes, it's not that you struggle to fall asleep, it's that a condition like sleep apnea affects the quality of sleep you get.

If you usually get seven or eight hours of sleep but still wake up tired, you might be waking yourself up at night without even knowing it. Or you might be a heavy snorer, which might also be affecting your quality of sleep.

Speak to your doctor if you are having this problem. They might first want to rule out other potential causes of fatigue like anemia. Still, if there are no other likely causes, a sleep study will confirm if you suffer from sleep apnea.

If you have sleep apnea, there are many remedies, from CPAP machines to surgery, that can help.

Practice Good Sleep Hygiene

Good sleep hygiene is a set of simple rules that make it more likely that you will get a good night's rest. These include:

- Not keeping your bedroom too warm or too cold.
- Removing electronic devices like televisions, phones, and tablets from your bedroom.
- Ensuring that there is adequate airflow in your room.
- Blocking out as much sound and light from your bedroom as possible.
- Trying to stick to roughly the same bedtime and morning alarm time.
- Avoid caffeine and alcohol for several hours before going to sleep.

Basically, to get good sleep, you need darkness, silence, and a comfortable bed.

Natural Sleep Aids

If you still struggle to nod off, you may need to try a natural sleep aid.

There are a variety available, including valerian root and melatonin. Some people also say that CBD helps them sleep, but that depends on what's available in your area.

Your doctor should be able to advise you on which sleep aids might work for you. None of these are narcotics, though, so they won't affect your mental health, and they aren't addictive.

Go to Sleep When You're Tired

Very often, we force ourselves to stay awake to watch another episode or finish an important project. Then, when we finally do go to bed, we can't fall asleep.

Pushing yourself when you're tired can make it harder to sleep, so try to plan your day so you can go to sleep when you feel tired.

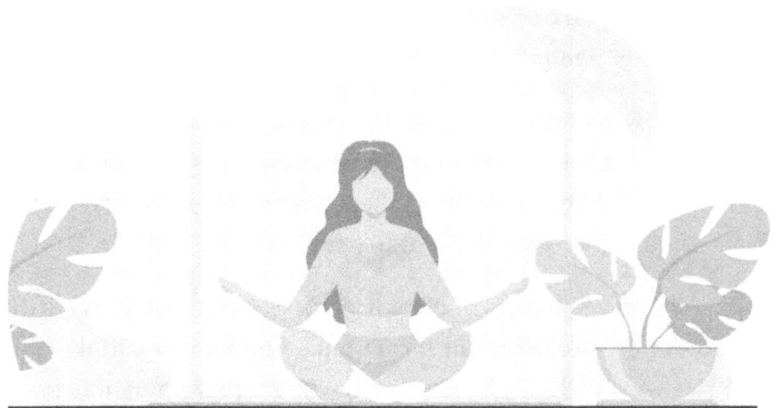

Banish the Stress!

Here's another one that is a lot easier said than done. People will tell you to destress, but it can be hard to figure out how to do that when you're in the thick of it. Stress releases a whole cocktail of chemicals, and this made sense when we were still living in caves and chasing our dinner with pointy sticks, but it doesn't really work now.

As you've seen, your metabolism is very much affected by chemicals, hormones, and other biological processes, so things that throw you out of whack are not good.

These practical tips can help.

Talk About It

Ever heard the saying, "a problem shared is a problem halved?" It's a cliché for a reason!

Even if you can't solve the problems that are causing you to be stressed, you can talk to someone about them, and that will make you feel a little better about it.

Talk to a family member or a friend. If you can't find one of those, find a helpline or chat room where you can share what's bothering you and talk to a stranger. Venting about things that are stressing us out is one of the best ways to release some of the pressure.

Facing your problems, giving them a name, and not burying them might not fix the problem, but it can make you realize that it's not the end of the world. You will still be here tomorrow, and it'll be a lot better if you're healthy and strong!

Give Yourself a Talking to

Another good way to deal with stress is to remind yourself that the things that seem monumental today probably won't matter in a year or two years.

Whatever is happening in your life that is stressing you out, you can get past it. Remember the question, "How do you eat an elephant?"

One bite at a time.

Spend some time working on a game plan to get you from where you are now to where you want to be. Break it all into small steps, and then take one after the other.

Other people can help you on your journey to health, weight loss, and wellness. Still, ultimately, it is you, your willpower, and determination that will determine your success. If you're always talking down to yourself and don't believe that you can change (or even that you want to), no amount of books, pep talks, or plans will help.

So, get your head in the game, commit, and get started!

. . .

Seek Help

If you are so stressed that it affects your eating habits, sleep, and life in general, it might be more serious than being a little stressed.

Prolonged, sustained stress can be dangerous in many ways, so if you feel like you've been overwhelmed for a long time, it's time to talk to your doctor or another professional.

There are treatments, including medications, which can help you to manage stress. Think of it as if it were any other medical condition. You wouldn't turn down heart medication or a cast on a broken leg. So don't deny yourself treatment for stress.

Take a Break!

One of the best ways to relieve stress is to get really good at doing nothing.

Yoga, meditation, or even something as simple as spending a whole day reading a book on the couch, are all good ways to give yourself a break from the stresses of the world.

You don't have to be "on" all the time. You can take a break, and you deserve one.

With all the demands of modern life, particularly if you have a job and a family, you not only deserve time off, but you also need to demand it. Block time out in your schedule that is just for you. Leave the house to get away from family demands. Turn your phone off after work on a Friday.

It's a good thing to be there for other people, but when it comes to your life and your stress levels, you have to be there for yourself too.

. . .

Be Realistic

If you're reading this book, it's very likely that your weight and health are some of the things that are causing you stress.

While it's good to pay attention to your health, it's not productive to get so stressed about it that you self-sabotage.

You need to accept that if you're out of shape, it probably took a while to get that way, and it will take some time to get back to where you want to be. Give yourself time, and remember that when you first start a new lifestyle plan, very often, you won't see results for a while.

Think of it as trying to pull a heavy object. First, you have to rock it a little to get it moving. Then you get it going ever so slowly, and eventually, it picks up speed and almost seems to move on its own. Your body is like that too. If it's been sitting in stasis for a while, it'll take a while to really get going, but if you stick to it, it will get going again.

Look out for small victories, and when they start happening, celebrate! If you're past the stage of rocking yourself out of being stuck, all you need to do is keep pulling, and you'll get to the free-wheeling stage soon enough!

Don't Compare

One of the worst things we do in life, in all areas, is to compare ourselves to other people.

Sure, there's a guy at work who eats burgers for lunch every day and still has a six-pack. Yes, your sister is five years older than you but looks like she could be on the cover of a magazine.

That's great for them, and hopefully, it will stay that way for them.

But if you're so busy wishing you could be like them, being jealous and envious, and feeling sorry for yourself, you're never going to have the time and energy to do the work that you need to do.

There will always be people who seem to have something easier than you do, but that's not always exactly how it is. Maybe those people have an eating disorder or some other condition that prevents them from gaining weight. Perhaps, when you aren't around, they only eat lettuce leaves, and they spend their nights in their basement doing aerobics videos.

The story you see on the surface is rarely the whole truth, and it's also absolutely irrelevant to you.

Ditch the Miracle Cures

When it comes to diet shakes, pills, and potions, none are actually proven to do anything.

Diet shakes usually taste terrible and are really just meals in liquid form. You can have tastier food (*and often healthier food*) with more variety for a fraction of the price.

Many diet drinks are basically just caffeine. Yes, caffeine helps to speed up your metabolism, but you can do that with a cup of coffee for a fraction of the price.

There is not a single diet product on the market that doesn't include the phrase "only effective with a calorie-controlled diet and exercise plan." You're going to do that anyway, so why spend a fortune on something that really does nothing?

If you rely on anything to help you on your way, look into a reputable calorie counting and exercise app. There are several on the market, and many are free. While they can't make you do the right things, they do help you track your progress, and it's a little like having a digital trainer you're accountable to. Nothing beats willpower, but if you can get a little help, take it.

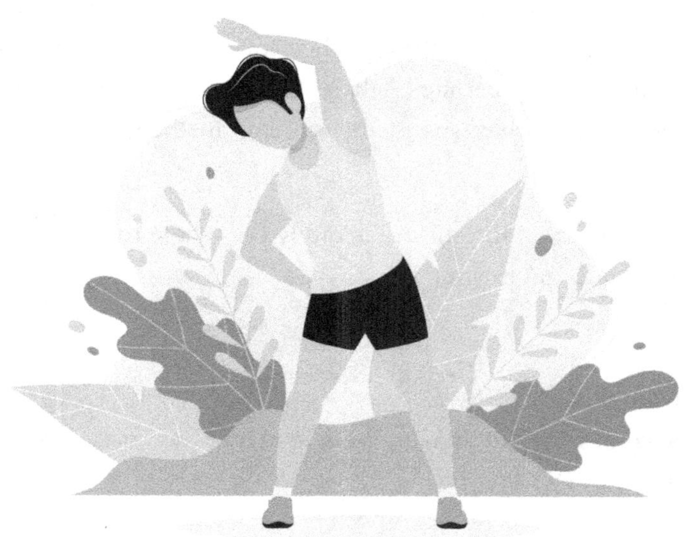

Exercise

Exercise is another big part of managing and improving your metabolism. Still, it can be hard to find the time and the motivation, so here are some ideas that might help:

- Find a sport that you love to play and join a local team. You don't have to be any good to have fun and have a great workout!
- Invest in an exercise system that connects you virtually with a trainer. If you don't physically have to leave your house to work out, there's no excuse!
- Spend more time doing activities you love. Dancing, ice

skating, cycling, hiking, climbing, and many more are great workouts!

- Walk more. Even if you have no time to go to the gym, you can always find time to walk. If you don't have to buy a lot of groceries and the store is within walking distance, take a backpack along and walk there. You'll get a great workout, and the weight of the groceries means you get a built-in strength workout!
- Be a good Samaritan. Offer to walk a neighbor's dog for them or clear the snow off an elderly person's driveway.
- Enlist a friend who also wants to get into shape to be your exercise buddy.
- Find exercise videos online and use them to try different kinds of workout.
- Take martial arts lessons.
- Invest in a set of weights and do a weight workout while you watch your favorite shows.
- Invest in an exercise bike or elliptical trainer and do a workout while you watch the news.
- Get a smartwatch, set a step goal, and make sure you hit it every day.
- Invest in a gaming system that includes motion detection. Then dance, play tennis, or box in your living room.
- Take your kids to the playground and join them on the monkey bars and swings. You'll be surprised how energetic kids actually are!
- Try a climbing wall.
- Join a water aerobics class at the local community center.
- Take a weekly walking tour around your city or commit to exploring one new park every week.
- If you find exercise dull, plug into your digital playlist, or listen to an audiobook while working out. You can even binge-watch series while you're working out. Whatever

> makes it easier to do and helps ensure that you do it is the right way!
>
> - Get competitive. If you find that winning is a motivator, get competitive! Sign up for a local park run or race your own times. Keep track of how far, how fast, or how much weight you can lift, and break your own records!

There are endless ways to get yourself moving. Very few of them require you to be in a gym, or even to buy special equipment or clothing.

When it comes to your metabolism, both cardio and weight or strength training are important. Cardio helps to burn calories that you eat, but building muscle raises your basal metabolic rate, so you can burn calories even when you're not doing anything.

You can find ways to do things you already love to do, and the more you like doing them, the easier it is to stick to them.

Hydrate

Up to 75% of people who live in the developed world are chronically dehydrated.

That's a very scary statistic.

Since we tend to confuse thirst with hunger, and since dehydration can affect our judgment, mood, and more, it's something that we definitely need to get a handle on.

Here are a few easy ways to make sure you get enough fluids to stay hydrated:

- Make sure that you drink a glass of water before every meal.
- Divide the day into two-hour segments and mark your water

bottle with "portion sizes." Set an alarm on your phone, and every time it goes off, drink one portion.

- Remember that while water is the holy grail for hydration, other fluids also count. Coffee and tea are good choices because they boost your metabolism, as are dairy and non-dairy milks. Don't get bored with water! Mix it up a little!
- Add some bubbles. Whether you buy commercial canned or bottled unsweetened sparkling water, or you invest in a carbonation system, fizzy water is more fun!
- If you plan to have alcohol, remember that it's a diuretic, so you need to alternate alcoholic drinks with water to stay hydrated.

We've already covered how being hydrated can have a marked impact on our metabolism. These tips are a good start on your road to being hydrated. Try them, and any others you might think up yourself.

Remember that fruits and vegetables also have a lot of liquid in them, so they also count towards your total intake.

Finally, when it comes to figuring out if you are dehydrated, there are a few ways to tell. One of the best is the color of your urine. If it's very dark, you're probably not getting enough fluids. It should be a very pale yellow. If you don't urinate four or more times a day, you might also be dehydrated.

Feeling fatigued even if you have had enough sleep is another sign of dehydration, as is dizziness and a dry mouth.

Chronic or severe dehydration can be a dangerous condition, so if you aren't getting enough water, start now! Your metabolism and your overall health will thank you!

Maintenance

Getting your metabolism back to where it should be is much like any other lifestyle change.

You will need to do more intense work to begin with, but once you've met your goals, you will be able to be a little more lenient with yourself. Once you reach the maintenance stage, you'll be able to add indulgences like dinners out or junk food on occasion to your lifestyle without throwing everything out of whack.

But you still have to make an effort, so here are some good rules when you reach the metabolism maintenance phase:

- Follow the 90/10 rule. If you do the right thing 90% of the time, you can cheat a little the other 10%.
- Get your family and friends on board with your lifestyle changes. It's well known that we tend to be like the people we spend the most time with. So, if you spend all your time with junk food eating couch potatoes, it's going to be very hard to stick to your lifestyle changes.
- Monitor your health. You don't have to obsess but pay attention to what the scale says and how your clothes fit. If you find yourself going in the wrong direction, you need to intensify your efforts again.
- Have regular medical checkups. There are all kinds of organs and glands involved in your metabolism, and if there's a problem with one of them, you will struggle to stay on top of it. Aside from being a good idea in general, knowing what's going on in your body will make a big difference to your long-term metabolic maintenance.
- Monitor your body fat. Even if you're relatively light, if you have a high proportion of body fat, you're going to have a sluggish metabolism. It's actually better to be a little heavier

with more muscle, and since muscle weighs more than fat, you might find that you don't look bigger, even if you weigh a little more. This is why weight alone is a poor indicator of health.

- Never stop learning. Science changes all the time. Things we believe to be true today might not be tomorrow, but that's just how science works. Get your information from reputable sources, and if the science changes, change your lifestyle to suit.

The good news is that even if getting your metabolism back on track is hard to get used to initially, by the time you've lived with these changes for a few weeks or months, they will become a habit. In turn, these habits will be solidified in your lifestyle.

Many times, the reason we gain more weight than we should is because it happens so slowly. We go up one size, and we think it's no big deal. Then, before we know it, we're up three sizes, and on the brink of needing a new wardrobe again.

Weight, health, and fitness are very often a matter of paying attention. When things aren't working the way they should, taking action before things get out of control is much easier than waiting.

But it's also never too late to take charge.

Good habits are easy to maintain too. Just keep doing what works!

**SLEEP IS THE MOST
IMPORTANT 'REPAIR'
MECHANISM OUR BODY
HAS, AND GETTING ENOUGH
OF IT WILL ENSURE YOU'RE
FEELING FIT AND ENERGIZED
THE NEXT DAY.**

- Jason Smith

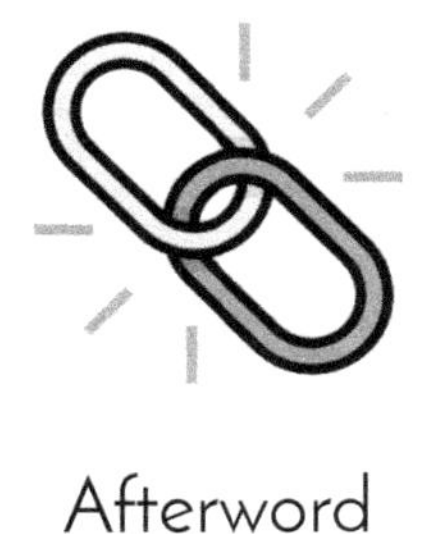

Afterword

I hope that this book has demystified the term "metabolism" and that you know the basics of how it works, what affects it, and what you can do to change yours.

Hopefully, you've also learned that sometimes, it's not something that you can control on your own. Many medical conditions can affect organs, glands, and processes, and may make it harder to lose weight and keep it off.

Your body, health, weight, and metabolism are all very complex and require a wide range of changes and tweaks to get into their best possible shape.

So, if you need to speak to your doctor to address an underlying problem, don't feel embarrassed. It's always a good idea to address medical issues before they cause too much trouble.

Metabolism is often seen as this mysterious force. We blame it when we get a little heavier. We envy people we believe have a faster metabolism, and we try to ignore that it changes as we get older.

But it's neither mysterious nor entirely out of our control.

This book gives you the tools to make changes that will impact your metabolism, but don't expect them to work overnight. In most cases, it takes many years to put on extra pounds, so it makes no sense that they will magically disappear overnight.

But if you make the changes, put in the work, and are consistent, you can do it.

Make changes when you notice that what you've been doing isn't working as well as it used to but remember that life is about more than obsessing about your waistline. If you're happy, healthy, and living your best life, you're doing it right!

There's no absolute right way to eat, work out or do anything else, and there's no one on the planet that gets it all right, all the time. The best we can do is use the information we have available and try to do our best most of the time.

As you've learned, though, starving yourself is not the answer. If you've been trying that approach, you may actually have slowed your metabolism down. But nothing is ever impossible to fix. It just takes a little work and the right approach.

So, don't beat yourself up if you've seen things here that you have been doing wrong. It's never too late to change the way you live, and you can start doing better things today.

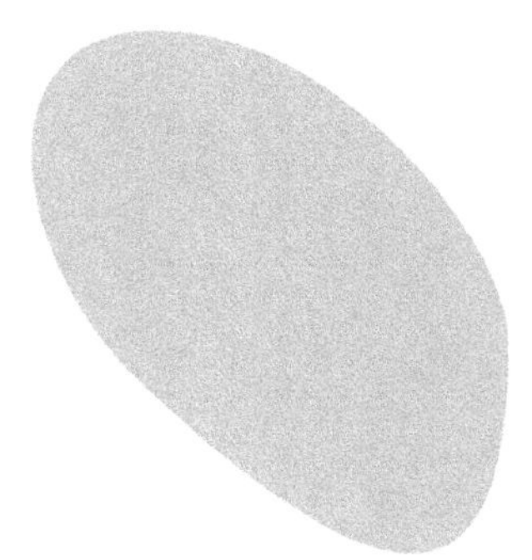

YOUR JOURNEY TO A
HEALTHIER WEIGHT IS NOT
A JOURNEY THAT YOU
START AND THEN GIVE UP.
IT IS A JOURNEY THAT YOU
ARE LIVING EVERY DAY FOR
THE REST OF YOUR LIFE.

– Thich Nhat Hanh

Thank You

Thank you for reading this book and allowing us to share our knowledge with you.

If you've enjoyed this book, please let us know by leaving an Amazon rating and a brief review! It only takes about 30 seconds, and it helps us compete against big publishing houses. It also helps other readers find my work!

Thank you for your time, and have an awesome day!

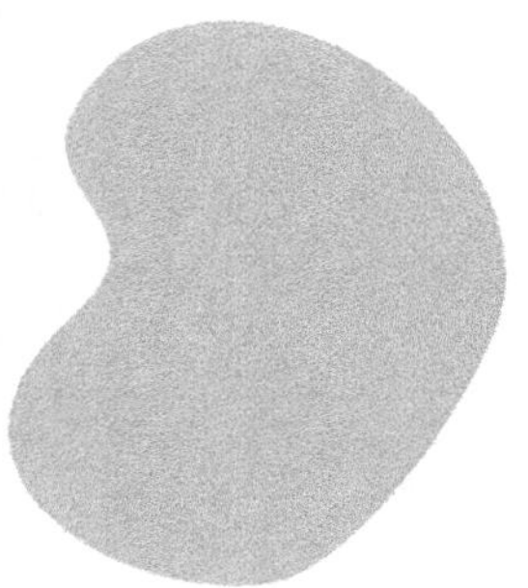

**BE DISCERNING ABOUT
THE FOODS YOU
CONSUME WITH A
GOAL OF NOURISHMENT,
NOT RESTRICTION.**

- Becca Shern

Resources

The good news about weight loss and health is that there's a lot of information out there. The bad news is that a lot of that information isn't 100% accurate.

The best way to ensure that the information you are getting is safe and reliable is to refer to trustworthy sources. University medical departments, research papers, and reputable, science-based websites are all excellent choices.

If anything seems to be designed to push you to purchase a product, there's a good chance it's not an entirely reliable source, so exercise caution. There are no shortcuts, no miracle pills, or potions.

Impact of stress on metabolism and energy balance

A study related to the connection between stress, energy and fitness, and metabolic rate.

https://www.sciencedirect.com/science/article/pii/S2352154616300183

The impact of stress on body function: A review

A broader look at the biological impact of stress on our health and wellness.

https://www.ncbi.nlm.nih.gov/pmc/articles/PMC5579396/

Interactions between sleep, stress, and metabolism: From physiological to pathological conditions

A study examining how stress and sleep affect metabolism and other bodily functions.

https://www.ncbi.nlm.nih.gov/pmc/articles/PMC4688585/

Yogurt consumption, weight change and risk of overweight/obesity: the SUN cohort study

A 2014 study into the relationship between yogurt consumption and weight

https://pubmed.ncbi.nlm.nih.gov/25001921/

Water-Induced Thermogenesis

Research into how drinking water can cause us to burn more calories.

https://academic.oup.com/jcem/article/88/12/6015/2661518

The impact of water intake on energy intake and weight status: a systematic review

How water impacts weight loss and gain in general.

https://www.ncbi.nlm.nih.gov/pmc/articles/PMC2929932/

Increasing muscle mass to improve metabolism.

A paper detailing the relationship between muscle mass and metabolic rate.

https://www.ncbi.nlm.nih.gov/pmc/articles/PMC3661116/

Sleep and Metabolism: An Overview

How sleep and metabolism are linked.

https://www.ncbi.nlm.nih.gov/pmc/articles/PMC2929498/

Lack of sleep affects fat metabolism.

A paper examining proof of the relationship between sleep and metabolism.

https://www.sciencedaily.com/releases/2019/09/190916114020.htm

Importance of Nutrients and Nutrient Metabolism on Human Health

A closer look at the metabolism of nutrients and our health.

https://www.ncbi.nlm.nih.gov/pmc/articles/PMC6020734/

Other Books By Brittney & Craig

- Liver Detox & Cleanse
- Gut Detox & Cleanse
- Carb Cycling Diet Plan & Cookbook